Conceptual Care Mapping

Case Studies for Improving Communication, Collaboration, Care

Barbara L. Yoost, MSN, RN, CNS, CNE, ANEF

Adjunct Professor
Division of Nursing
Notre Dame College
South Euclid, Ohio

Lynne R. Crawford, MSN, RN, MBA, CNE

Retired Faculty
College of Nursing
Kent State University
Kent, Ohio

ELSEVIER

ELSEVIER

3251 Riverport Lane
St. Louis, Missouri 63043

Library of Congress Cataloging-in-Publication Data
Names: Yoost, Barbara L., author. | Crawford, Lynne R., author.
Title: Conceptual care mapping / Barbara L. Yoost, Lynne R. Crawford.
Description: Philadelphia, PA : Elsevier, [2018] | Includes bibliographical
    references.
Identifiers: LCCN 2016048598 | ISBN 9780323480376 (pbk. : alk. paper)
Subjects: | MESH: Education, Nursing--methods | Nursing Process | Concept
    Formation | Problem Solving | Patient-Centered Care | Evidence-Based
    Nursing--education | Case Reports
Classification: LCC RT71 | NLM WY 18 | DDC 610.73071--dc23 LC record available at https://lccn.loc.
gov/2016048598

Executive Content Strategist: Tamara Myers
Content Development Manager: Lisa Newton
Senior Content Development Specialist: Laura Selkirk
Publishing Services Manager: Jeff Patterson
Senior Project Manager: Tracey Schriefer
Design Direction: Amy Buxton

Printed in Canada

Last digit is the print number: 9   8   7   6   5   4   3   2   1

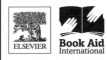

We dedicate this book to our students, patients, and colleagues.

*To our students who were the motivation behind developing the **Conceptual Care Map**: an active learning tool that facilitates thorough collection, analysis, and synthesis of data in the clinical, lab, or classroom setting while contributing to safer patient-centered care. Thank you for your inspiration.*

To our patients who provide unlimited opportunities for student learning and professional growth. Thank you for the privilege of caring for you.

*To our colleagues who recognize the value of the **Conceptual Care Map** and case-based active learning across the curriculum. Thank you for your support and your commitment to transformative nursing education.*

Reviewers

Shawnadine K. Becenti, RN, MSN
Lecturer, Nursing
University of New Mexico-Gallup
Gallup, New Mexico

Susan Frances Camasi, RN, MSN, LRN
Assistant Professor, School of Nursing
University of Alaska Anchorage
Anchorage, Alaska

Janice M. Crabill, PhD, RN
Associate Professor, Nursing
Northwest Nazarene University
Nampa, Idaho

Marci L. Dial, DNP, MSN, BSN, ARNP, NP-C, RN-BC, CHSE, LNC
Professor of Nursing, Department of Nursing
Valencia College
Orlando, Florida

Katrina Dielman, MS, RN
Clinical Instructor, Undergraduate Nursing Program
Oregon Health and Science University
La Grande, Oregon

Christina Flint, RN, MSN, MBA
Assistant Professor of Nursing
University of Indianapolis
Indianapolis, Indiana

Mariann M. Harding, PhD, RN, CNE
Associate Professor of Nursing
Kent State University Tuscarawas
New Philadelphia, Ohio

Dorothy Kinley, RN, MS, CMSRN
Assistant Professor, School of Nursing
University of Alaska Anchorage
Anchorage, Alaska

Janis Longfield McMillan, MSN, RN, CNE
Associate Clinical Professor, School of Nursing
Northern Arizona University
Flagstaff, Arizona

Sandra Gayle Nadelson, RN, MSN, MSEd,PhD, CNE
Program Director, Nursing and Health Professions
Utah State University
Logan, Utah

Kristie Stephens, RN, PHN, MSN
Dean, School of Nursing
Simpson University
Redding, California

Brenda Trigg, DNP, GNP, CNE, RN
Professor of Nursing, Department Chair
Southern Arkansas University
Magnolia, Arkansas

Rachelle K. White, BSN, RN, CWON
Assistant Nursing Instructor, School of Nursing
University of Alaska Anchorage
Anchorage, Alaska

Laura C. Williams, MSN, CNS, ONC, CCNS
Orthopedic Clinical Nurse Specialist
Center for Nursing Research and Advanced
   Nursing Practice
Orlando Health
Orlando, Florida

Preface

Conceptual Care Mapping: Case Studies for Improving Communication, Collaboration, and Care is an active learning and performance assessment resource for students that provides transformative nursing education, connecting theory and practice. While addressing the issues of care, interprofessional collaboration, effective communication, and critical thinking, the text supports the advancement of clinical judgment skills in student nurses and prepares them to provide more patient-centered, evidence-based care. Prelicensure Quality and Safety Education for Nurses (QSEN) and National Academy of Medicine (formerly the IOM) competencies are explored throughout the book.

The first five chapters of *Conceptual Care Mapping: Case Studies for Improving Communication, Collaboration, and Care* provide foundational information to reinforce what is being learned in clinical nursing courses. Chapter 1 introduces the student to the Conceptual Care Map (CCM), which mimics the electronic health record (EHR) and care planning approaches of most health care facilities. The CCM tool was developed 10 years ago by the authors to identify student competency surrounding the collection, analysis, and synthesis of patient data, and evidence-based, patient-centered care. Conceptual Care Mapping has been adopted by many programs across the country and around the world as an effective tool for the organization of patient data, care planning, and evaluation of student outcomes.

Conceptual Care Map Creator software is available as an Evolve resource for online care plan development and submission, or blank CCM forms can be printed out for use in various settings. Appendix B contains a *Conceptual Care Map Submission Checklist* that allows students to take responsibility for the thorough completion of their work. The CCM can replace or supplement traditional care plans in the academic setting and/or be used in the clinical setting as a daily work sheet and then developed into an assignment for evaluation of clinical knowledge and judgment. The CCM combined with Case Studies 1 through 30 provides for active learning in the classroom, skills, or simulation lab.

A Conceptual Care Map Grading Rubric is available online as an assessment tool to ensure grading consistency. This is especially helpful when multiple instructors, both seasoned and novice, are involved in evaluation. The grading rubric can be adapted for scoring according to each program's curriculum needs.

Chapters 2 through 5 provide a brief overview of assessment, communication, collaboration, and critical thinking. Key strategies for patient assessment, data validation, and documentation are highlighted. Communication skills critical to patient safety and effective care are reviewed, as well as handoff communication. Interprofessional collaboration and delegation strategies and expectations are presented to enhance student development in these essential areas of professional practice. To emphasize the integration of evidence-based practice into student care planning, the crucial aspects of critical thinking, its components, and methods for improvement are addressed.

The thirty case studies, presented as patient assignments, in *Conceptual Care Mapping: Case Studies for Improving Communication, Collaboration, and Care*, focus student attention on comprehensive patient care. The cases build from simple to complex, beginning with pneumonia and progressing to the fundamental aspects of caring for a patient with sepsis. Students are asked to address patient safety concerns, including medication administration, diagnostic study analysis, interdisciplinary care, psychomotor skills, crisis intervention, evidence-based interventions, transfer handoffs, and more, while "caring" and responding to patient changes throughout evolving case studies. Answer keys for each odd numbered case study (1, 3, 5, etc.) are available immediately to students online on Evolve. Answer keys for even numbered case studies are available to students at the discretion of faculty to allow for individual, graded performance assessment and student evaluation.

In the past 10 years, Conceptual Care Mapping has proven to have a significant impact on student competency and safe, patient-centered care. We are excited to share this transformative learning and assessment resource with nursing students and faculty colleagues everywhere.

Barbara L. Yoost, MSN, RN, CNS, CNE, ANEF
Lynne R. Crawford, MSN, RN, MBA, CNE

Contents

1

Introduction to Conceptual Care Mapping

Learning Outcomes

Comprehension of this chapter's content will provide students with the ability to:

LO 1.1   Describe how to use the conceptual care map for organization and synthesis of patient data.

LO 1.2   Develop a patient-centered care plan using the nursing process within the conceptual care map.

The key to providing safe, individualized patient-centered care is for the nurse to be able to identify patient problems or concerns, prioritize them, and implement evidence-based interventions that are acceptable to the patient or the patient's guardian. Nursing practice requires high-level critical thinking and clinical judgments that may result in improved quality of life for, injury to, or death of a patient. Clinical decision making may involve the action of one nurse or an entire team of health care professionals. In every situation, the nurse must be capable of understanding the complexities of patient care and responding quickly with the appropriate interventions.

Conceptual care mapping combines two educational strategies: the concept map and the nursing process. Conceptual care mapping mimics the thought process of the professional nurse, guides patient care, and provides a tool for evaluation. Using the conceptual care map (CCM) increases a student's ability to accurately collect, analyze, and synthesize patient data. Conceptual care mapping supports both students and nurses to practice at their highest level of professional ability. Whether using the CCM with a case study patient or in clinical practice, it helps to organize, plan, and implement safe, evidence-based, patient-centered care.

Collecting and Synthesizing Data   LO 1.1

Collecting patient data often requires obtaining information from a patient's electronic health record (EHR) and members of the health care team, interviewing the patient, family members, friends, or care providers, and completing either a focused or complete patient physical assessment. All of this data is organized in the first of two major sections of the CCM, which is divided into seven subsections. Fig. 1.1 shows the data organization and synthesis section of the CCM. Note that each subsection provides space to document patient information and guides the process of gathering and organizing the data.

Demographic and Anthropometric Data

Data collection starts with identifying basic information for a patient, including age, gender, admission date, and religion. This information can be obtained by reviewing the patient's EHR, and then verified by checking with the patient or guardian. The middle top subsection of the data collection area provides space for recording this information. In addition, this subsection holds anthropometric data such as the patient's height and weight, and basic orders including code status, diet, and activity. Note that listing allergies and Braden score findings will require interaction and assessment by the nurse before documentation. Fig. 1.2 is an example of a completed demographic and anthropometric subsection of the CCM. Remember that some of this information will change throughout a patient's hospitalization, and at times even within hours depending on the patient's condition. So, be prepared to edit and analyze the changes and how they impact patient care.

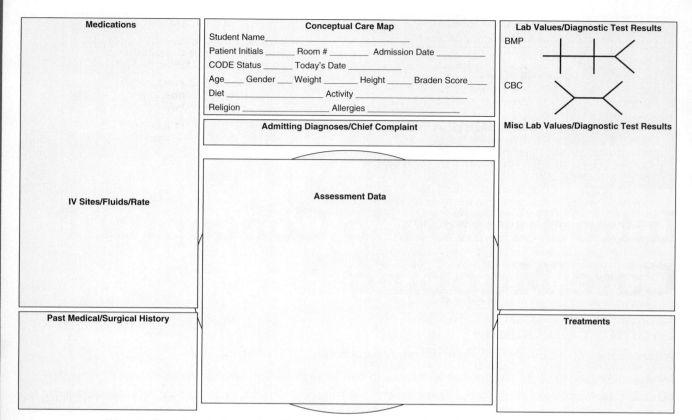

FIG. 1.1 The data collection section of the Conceptual Care Map (CCM) provides an organizational framework for documenting patient information that must be analyzed and synthesized before planning care.

Conceptual Care Map

Student Name_____

Patient Initials _M.P._ Room # _321_ Admission Date _12/29/18_

CODE Status _Full_ Today's Date _12/30/18_

Age _76_ Gender _M_ Weight _84.4 kg (186 lb)_ Height _149.8 cm (59 in)_ Braden Score _20_

Diet _2000 mg Na diet_ Activity _Up with assistance_

Religion _Presbyterian_ Allergies _Penicillin_

FIG. 1.2 Initial patient data is recorded in the demographic and anthropometric subsection.

Admitting Diagnosis/Chief Complaint and Assessment Data

Collecting a comprehensive body of relevant patient data is crucial before identifying the needs of patients and providing individualized, competent care. After documenting initial baseline demographic and anthropometric data, the nurse must record relevant assessment data over a period of time. The middle subsections of the CCM (Fig. 1.3) are the areas used to begin documentation. Here the nurse records the patient's admitting diagnoses and/or chief complaint. A patient may be admitted with more than one medical diagnosis, making it important to list them all in this subsection of the CCM. Listening to the patient and identifying the patient's chief complaint is also helpful in guiding patient-centered care. For instance, a patient may be admitted with medical diagnoses of

heart failure and *aortic stenosis* with a chief complaint of *shortness of breath.*

The large assessment subsection accommodates both subjective and objective patient data and information over time. In this section, results of either a focused or complete physical assessment are recorded as well as cultural, emotional, sexual, and spiritual information collected or shared by the patient or guardian (see Chapter 2 for detailed information on assessment techniques and strategies).

Subjective data are spoken information or symptoms that often cannot be authenticated. Subjective data are best documented in quotes to indicate verbatim statements. Statements may include descriptions of feeling dizzy or ill, emotions, concerns, and other types of knowledge that may or may not be validated objectively. For example, if a patient is experiencing chest pain and says, "It feels like an elephant is standing on my chest,"

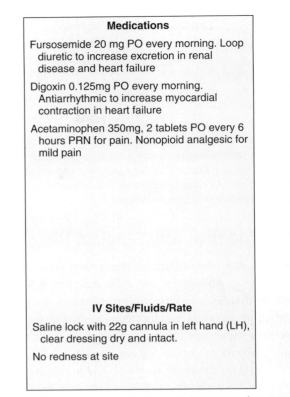

Admitting Diagnoses/Chief Complaint

Heart failure and aortic stenosis/shortness of breath

Assessment Data

Vital signs:T 37.1° C (98.8° F), P 110 and regular, R 24 and labored, BP 130/82; pulse oximetry 94% on 2 L of O_2 via nasal cannula.

Denies pain but states, "I felt like I couldn't get enough air at home. I was winded just walking around the house and I feel so tired all the time." Alert and oriented x4. Neuro exam is within normal limits (WNL). Speech is clear and hearing is normal.

Skin is warm to touch. Crackles heard in all lung fields bilaterally. Systolic murmur noted on auscultation of the heart. No pulse deficit. Peripheral pulses are palpable with no edema noted. Abdomen soft and nontender with BS present in all 4 quadrants. Musculoskeletal exam is WNL.

I&O: 200 mL juice with breakfast and 50 mL of water with medications. Voided in urinal, 180 mL of clear amber urine.

Married for 52 years and states, "My wife will be in to see me this afternoon." Patient states that his wife attends a Presbyterian church but he doesn't go very often.

FIG. 1.3 Detailed patient assessment information provides critical insight into a patient's condition, the patient's stability, and factors that help to determine and guide care.

Box 1.1 Examples of Subjective and Objective Patient Data

Subjective Data	Objective Data
"I didn't get much sleep last night."	BP-124/62
"I've had diabetes since I was 10 years old."	WBC-6700
"I am scared about starting chemotherapy tomorrow."	Apical pulse-74 and regular
"My pain is mostly in my hip, although it radiates to my lower back sometimes, too."	Urine-cloudy, slightly pink tinged without clots
	Gait steady while ambulating independently

BP, Blood pressure; *WBC*, white blood cell count.

---

the nurse should include the patient's statement in his or her medical record.

Objective data, also referred to as signs, can be measured or observed. The nurse's senses of sight, hearing, touch, and smell are used to collect objective data. Objective assessment data are acquired through observation, physical examination, and analysis of laboratory and diagnostic test results. Examples of objective data are blood pressure readings, pulse measurement, and hemoglobin levels; any information that can be compared with established norms (Box 1.1).

Recording sequential vital signs allows easy comparison and the rapid evaluation of any changes in patient health status. Additional information that can guide or provide

---

Medications

Fursosemide 20 mg PO every morning. Loop diuretic to increase excretion in renal disease and heart failure

Digoxin 0.125mg PO every morning. Antiarrhythmic to increase myocardial contraction in heart failure

Acetaminophen 350mg, 2 tablets PO every 6 hours PRN for pain. Nonopioid analgesic for mild pain

IV Sites/Fluids/Rate

Saline lock with 22g cannula in left hand (LH), clear dressing dry and intact.

No redness at site

FIG. 1.4 Listing thorough medication, and intravenous therapy and site information is important for providing safe patient care and transferring critical information to other health care team members.

---

insight into the patient's condition should also be included in the assessment subsection.

Medications and Intravenous Therapy Information

Medication information is listed in the next subsection to the left. Listed are current medication orders, including all prescription and over-the-counter medications, and any vitamins or herbs prescribed by the patient's primary care provider (physician or nurse practitioner). In addition to listing the complete order including dose, route, and time/frequency of administration, the classification of the medication and the reason the patient is receiving the medication is recorded on the CCM. This process serves to reinforce the student's medication knowledge and document an understanding of the relevancy of each medication to the patient's current condition.

Primary intravenous (IV) therapy information is recorded at the bottom of the medication subsection. The type and rate of primary IV solutions are listed here. Assessment findings for each IV site, including the type (saline lock, central line, peripherally inserted central catheter [PICC], arteriovenous [AV] fistula), size of the cannula (16g, 22g, 25g), location, appearance, type of dressing, its condition, and whether the dressing includes the initials of the nurse who applied it are recorded for reference (Fig. 1.4).

FIG. 1.5 Documenting additional medical conditions for which the patient is not hospitalized or seeking treatment, and recording surgical procedures with dates of occurrence provide a better picture of the patient's overall health status for care planning.

Past Medical and Surgical History

In the lower left subsection, the patient's past medical diagnoses and surgeries are recorded (Fig. 1.5). These may be dramatically different or related to the patient's admitting diagnosis or chief complaint. For instance, a patient with an admitting diagnosis of heart failure may have a history of chronic kidney disease (CKD), making it essential for the nurse to note CKD in this subsection. Additional preexisting conditions and past surgeries, with dates of their occurrence, are also recorded here. Gathering this information is vitally important for gaining an overall picture of the patient's wellness and treatment challenges. Although a patient may be admitted with just one medical diagnosis, the nurse must plan care to address each need or problem of the patient, some of which may be multifaceted.

It may be possible to obtain initial history information by reviewing a patient's EHR. However, it is essential to speak directly to the patient or the patient's guardian to verify all medical record information. Through the use of both open- and closed-ended questions the nurse can obtain additional data during the health history interview. Additional information on communication is available in Chapter 3.

Laboratory Values and Diagnostic Test Results

To identify potential problems and evaluate a patient's condition, the nurse must be aware of and monitor the patient's laboratory (lab) and diagnostic test results. Examples of these include complete blood counts (CBC), basic metabolic panel (BMP), urine and stool cultures, x-rays, computerized axial tomography (CAT), bone, positron emission tomography (PET), and magnetic resonance imaging (MRI) scans, and ultrasound findings. The patient's lab results from the BMP and CBC are recorded in the lab skeleton provided in the upper right subsection of the CCM (Fig. 1.6). This type of lab skeleton is a standardized charting form used by health care practitioners around the world. Within the BMP lab skeleton, results for sodium (Na^+), chloride (Cl^-), and blood urea nitrogen

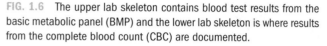

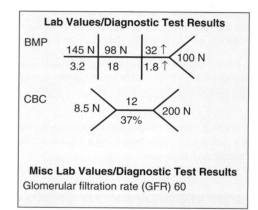

FIG. 1.6 The upper lab skeleton contains blood test results from the basic metabolic panel (BMP) and the lower lab skeleton is where results from the complete blood count (CBC) are documented.

FIG. 1.7 Pertinent lab results not included in lab skeleton are recorded in the Misc Lab values section of the Conceptual Care Map (CCM).

(BUN) are recorded from left to right on the top, with levels of potassium (K^+), carbon dioxide (CO_2), and creatinine documented along the bottom. The patient's blood glucose level is listed to the far right. Within the CBC lab skeleton, the patient's white blood cell (WBC) count is noted on the left, hemoglobin (Hgb) is recorded immediately above hematocrit (Hct), and platelets (Plt) are documented to the right. After each lab result is in place, students need to identify if the lab finding is normal (N), high (↑), or low (↓) by placing the corresponding symbol next to each result or by selecting the appropriate symbol from the pull down box below each finding in the *Conceptual Care Map Creator*.

Miscellaneous Laboratory Values

When a patient's lab results include values from tests not included in the lab skeletons, those findings are placed in the miscellaneous lab value section, followed by an indication of their relationship to normal (Fig. 1.7). When a lab result is outside of the normal range and marked with an ↑ or ↓, the student must note the normal range in parentheses in the miscellaneous lab values area with a brief explanation for the abnormal finding. For instance, if a patient with heart failure is placed on a loop diuretic, such as furosemide to reduce fluid retention, and the patient's potassium level is found to be below normal, the student should record the normal range for potassium in the miscellaneous lab value area followed by a statement like, "excess secretion of K^+ secondary (2°) to taking loop diuretic"

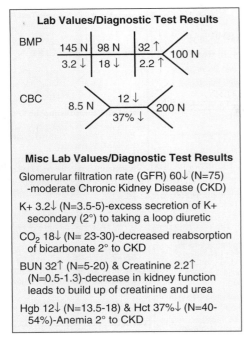

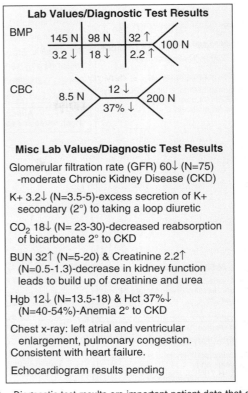

FIG. 1.8 Making note of the normal range for lab values that are high or low, and stating the probable cause for each reinforces knowledge of expected outcomes and demonstrates critical thinking skills.

(Fig. 1.8). Making this notation reinforces the student's knowledge base of normal lab values and the side effects of loop diuretics. It also demonstrates student competency and understanding when faculty evaluates the student's work.

Diagnostic Test Results

In addition to miscellaneous lab values, other diagnostic test results are documented in the lower area of this subsection. The name of each diagnostic test should be recorded indicating if the results are normal or abnormal, and if abnormal, followed by a brief explanation from the findings of the pathologist or radiologist. For example, if a patient in heart failure has a chest x-ray that indicates fluid retention in both lungs, this information should be noted under the diagnostic test results area as shown in Fig. 1.9.

Treatments

The bottom right subsection is the area of the CCM in which patient treatments are recorded. The treatments to list are nursing orders or orders of the patient's primary care provider (PCP). These may include treatments performed by a variety of health care team members including, but not limited to a nurse, respiratory therapist, social worker, physical therapist, dietitian, speech therapist, or patient (Fig. 1.10). Examples of treatments are vital signs every 4 (q4) hours, coughing and deep breathing every 2 (q2) hours, intake and output every (I&O q) shift, sequential compression device (SCD), cardiac rehabilitation three times a week after discharge, swallow test, dietary consult, extended care facility referral, or incentive spirometry every 1 (q1) hour while awake. When

FIG. 1.9 Diagnostic test results are important patient data that contribute vital information to the development of comprehensive treatment plans.

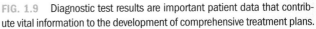

Treatments
Strict I&O q shift
Daily weights
Fluid restrictions 1800 mL/day
2000 mg sodium diet
O₂ via nasal cannula at 2L/hr
Vital signs q4h
Sequential compression devices (SCDs) when in bed
Up with assistance
Fall precautions
Coughing and deep breathing q 2 hours while awake
Incentive spirometry q 1 hour while awake
Cardiac rehab 3 times per week after discharge
Dietary consult

FIG. 1.10 Treatments requiring the intervention of various health care team members are listed for reference during patient care.

reviewing this list, it becomes obvious that many different people may be involved in patient care necessitating effective collaboration by the nurse with each member of the health care team. Additional information to facilitate effective interprofessional collaboration is found in Chapter 4.

Related Patient Data

Student understanding of the interrelatedness of patient information requires: (1) basic knowledge of the pathophysiology associated with each of the patient's problems,

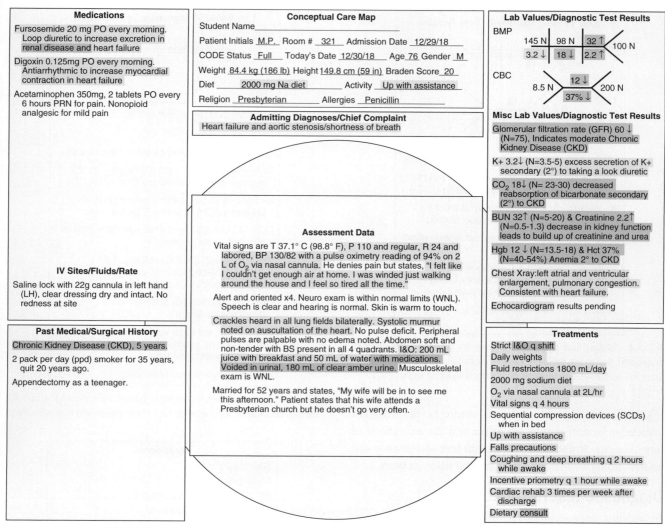

Medications

Fursosemide 20 mg PO every morning. Loop diuretic to increase excretion in renal disease and heart failure

Digoxin 0.125mg PO every morning. Antiarrhythmic to increase myocardial contraction in heart failure

Acetaminophen 350mg, 2 tablets PO every 6 hours PRN for pain. Nonopioid analgesic for mild pain

IV Sites/Fluids/Rate

Saline lock with 22g cannula in left hand (LH), clear dressing dry and intact. No redness at site

Past Medical/Surgical History

Chronic Kidney Disease (CKD), 5 years.

2 pack per day (ppd) smoker for 35 years, quit 20 years ago.

Appendectomy as a teenager.

Conceptual Care Map

Student Name_____

Patient Initials _M.P._ Room # _321_ Admission Date _12/29/18_

CODE Status _Full_ Today's Date _12/30/18_ Age _76_ Gender _M_

Weight _84.4 kg (186 lb)_ Height _149.8 cm (59 in)_ Braden Score _20_

Diet _____2000 mg Na diet_____ Activity ___Up with assistance___

Religion _Presbyterian_ Allergies _Penicillin_

Admitting Diagnoses/Chief Complaint
Heart failure and aortic stenosis/shortness of breath

Assessment Data

Vital signs are T 37.1° C (98.8° F), P 110 and regular, R 24 and labored, BP 130/82 with a pulse oximetry reading of 94% on 2 L of O_2 via nasal cannula. He denies pain but states, "I felt like I couldn't get enough air at home. I was winded just walking around the house and I feel so tired all the time."

Alert and oriented x4. Neuro exam is within normal limits (WNL). Speech is clear and hearing is normal. Skin is warm to touch.

Crackles heard in all lung fields bilaterally. Systolic murmur noted on auscultation of the heart. No pulse deficit. Peripheral pulses are palpable with no edema noted. Abdomen soft and non-tender with BS present in all 4 quadrants. I&O: 200 mL juice with breakfast and 50 mL of water with medications. Voided in urinal, 180 mL of clear amber urine. Musculoskeletal exam is WNL.

Married for 52 years and states, "My wife will be in to see me this afternoon." Patient states that his wife attends a Presbyterian church but he doesn't go very often.

Lab Values/Diagnostic Test Results

BMP

145 N 98 N 32 ↑ 100 N
3.2 ↓ 18 ↓ 2.2 ↑

CBC

8.5 N 12 ↓ 200 N
37% ↓

Misc Lab Values/Diagnostic Test Results

Glomerular filtration rate (GFR) 60 ↓ (N=75), Indicates moderate Chronic Kidney Disease (CKD)

K+ 3.2↓ (N=3.5-5) excess secretion of K+ secondary (2°) to taking a look diuretic

CO_2 18↓ (N= 23-30) decreased reabsorption of bicarbonate secondary (2°) to CKD

BUN 32↑ (N=5-20) & Creatinine 2.2↑ (N=0.5-1.3) decrease in kidney function leads to build up of creatinine and urea

Hgb 12 ↓ (N=13.5-18) & Hct 37% (N=40-54%) Anemia 2° to CKD

Chest Xray:left atrial and ventricular enlargement, pulmonary congestion. Consistent with heart failure.

Echocardiogram results pending

Treatments

Strict I&O q shift

Daily weights

Fluid restrictions 1800 mL/day

2000 mg sodium diet

O_2 via nasal cannula at 2L/hr

Vital signs q 4 hours

Sequential compression devices (SCDs) when in bed

Up with assistance

Falls precautions

Coughing and deep breathing q 2 hours while awake

Incentive priometry q 1 hour while awake

Cardiac rehab 3 times per week after discharge

Dietary consult

FIG. 1.11 Linkages among assessment data can be shown by highlighting related patient information.

and (2) synthesis of the data collected and documented. Comprehension of the complexity of a patient's condition is demonstrated on the CCM by highlighting patient information that is related. The best strategy to begin the process of synthesizing data is to consider the patient's admitting diagnoses, chief complaint, past medical conditions, and surgeries one at a time. Then proceed to consider the patient's signs and symptoms, prescribed medications, lab and diagnostic test results, and treatments, and look for their relatedness. Finally, highlight all of the related data to show their connection. For example, if the patient's admitting diagnosis is heart failure (HF), recall or look up the pathophysiology of HF, look at each of the subsections of the CCM for related information, then begin to highlight each piece of data that is associated with another. After highlighting data related to the admitting diagnoses, move on to link data related to other problems or concerns such as a patient's medical history of CKD.

Each connection is marked in a different color of highlighting to acknowledge that specific relationship (Fig. 1.11). When a piece of assessment information is related to one or more diagnosis or condition, it can be highlighted in more than one color. Highlighting related patient data demonstrates an understanding of the rationale for the patient's orders and treatments, and facilitates the development of a patient-centered care plan.

Developing an Individualized Plan of Care LO 1.2

The first seven subsections of the CCM contain patient information gathered during the assessment step of the nursing process. The second major section of the CCM continues with the identification of patient problems, potential problems, or responses to a problem or patient concern that represent the nursing diagnosis or analysis step of the nursing process (Fig. 1.12). When related patient data is highlighted, it forms a cluster of patient information that supports the nursing diagnosis or patient problem from which planning and goal setting emerges, interventions are formulated, and evaluation of patient outcomes are determined.

Primary Nursing Diagnosis	Nursing Diagnosis 2	Nursing Diagnosis 3
Supporting Data	Supporting Data	Supporting Data
STG/NOC	STG/NOC	STG/NOC
Interventions/NIC with Rationale	Interventions/NIC with Rationale	Interventions/NIC with Rationale
Rationale Citation/EBP	Rationale Citation/EBP	Rationale Citation/EBP
Evaluation	Evaluation	Evaluation

FIG. 1.12　The nursing process section of the Conceptual Care Map (CCM) provides the framework in which to develop a patient-centered plan of care.

Nursing Diagnosis or Problem Identification

Nursing diagnosis is the second step of the nursing process. Formulation of nursing diagnoses follows patient data collection and involves the analysis and clustering of related assessment information. If related patient information has been properly highlighted, each cluster of data becomes evidence to corroborate a nursing diagnosis or problem.

The CCM supports the use of official nursing diagnosis terminology, however, if an institution does not use NANDA-I or the International Classification for Nursing Practice (ICNP), patient problems rather than nursing diagnoses can be recorded in this area. Regardless of whether or not nursing diagnoses or problems are noted, each is followed by a brief statement indicating its physiologic or psychosocial etiology (underlying cause), and/or a cluster or list of associated data taken directly from the assessment information. The cluster of patient information serves to verify the existence of the identified patient

problem or potential problem. The nursing diagnosis or patient problem is highlighted in the color corresponding to the cluster of its supporting data recorded in the first section of the CCM. Fig. 1.13 demonstrates two different methods of completing the nursing diagnosis or problem identification step of the nursing process within the CCM. Once each nursing diagnosis or problem is formulated, the planning step of the nursing process begins in which each nursing diagnosis or problem is prioritized and patient outcome goals are written.

Planning

The planning phase of the nursing process begins with prioritizing patient problems according to the urgency with which each needs to be addressed. The patient's most crucial concern is listed in column one of the care planning section of the CCM, followed by subsequent nursing diagnoses or problems. Priorities can be determined using a variety of resources, including *Maslow's Hierarchy of Needs* or the ABC's (airway, breathing, circulation) of

Primary Nursing Diagnosis	Primary Patient Problem
Decreased cardiac output related to altered myocardial contractility as evidenced by…	Poor cardiac muscle function due to decreased myocardial contractility
Supporting Data P 110 and regular; Crackles heard in all lung fields bilaterally; Systolic murmur noted on auscultation of the heart; Chest x-ray: left atrial and ventricular enlargement, pulmonary congestion	**Supporting Data** P 110 and regular; Crackles heard in all lung fields bilaterally; Systolic murmur noted on auscultation of the heart; Chest x-ray: left atrial and ventricular enlargement, pulmonary congestion

FIG. 1.13 The nursing diagnosis and supporting data sections of the Conceptual Care Map (CCM) can be completed using NANDA-I or International Classification for Nursing Practice (ICNP) terminology, or problem identification.

life support in the health care setting. For each nursing diagnosis or problem, short-term and long-term goals and outcome indicators are formulated in collaboration with the patient and/or family members and care providers. Goals must be patient focused, realistic, and measureable. If Nursing Outcome Classifications (NOC) are used by an institution, the outcome indicator is noted next to the outcome. Following the determination of goals and outcome criterion, the nurse lists interventions that are evidence-based and acceptable to the patient to address each problem. If Nursing Intervention Classifications (NIC) are used, the exact terminology of the intervention is listed.

In the CCM, goals are noted in the Short Term Goal/Nursing Outcome Classification (STG/NOC) section and interventions are listed in the Interventions/NIC with Rationale section. A rationale is placed next to each intervention and the source for each rationale is documented in the Rationale Citation/EBP area (Fig. 1.14). To develop a patient-centered plan of care, it is vital to involve the patient and sometimes family members or other caregivers in the process of development. Evidence-based practice (EBP) includes (1) the best possible evidence, (2) clinical expertise of the nurse and other health care team members, (3) patient values and needs, and (4) cost-effectiveness (Yoost and Crawford, 2016).

Resources are available to students and nurses to assist in the identification of nursing diagnoses, goals and outcomes (NOC), and interventions (NIC). Appendix A contains NANDA-I nursing diagnosis labels and their definitions. Many additional online or text resources include definitions for nursing diagnoses, example goal statements or outcomes, and interventions with rationales needed to complete the CCM and develop a patient-centered plan of care. Some of the available resources are listed in Box 1.2.

Implementation and Evaluation

Carrying out the interventions determined within the planning stage may encompass a variety of actions

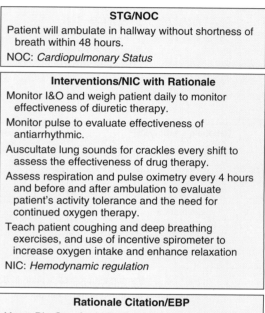

STG/NOC
Patient will ambulate in hallway without shortness of breath within 48 hours. NOC: *Cardiopulmonary Status*

Interventions/NIC with Rationale
Monitor I&O and weigh patient daily to monitor effectiveness of diuretic therapy. Monitor pulse to evaluate effectiveness of antiarrhythmic. Auscultate lung sounds for crackles every shift to assess the effectiveness of drug therapy. Assess respiration and pulse oximetry every 4 hours and before and after ambulation to evaluate patient's activity tolerance and the need for continued oxygen therapy. Teach patient coughing and deep breathing exercises, and use of incentive spirometer to increase oxygen intake and enhance relaxation NIC: *Hemodynamic regulation*

Rationale Citation/EBP
Yoost BL, Crawford LR. *Fundamentals of nursing: Active learning for collaborative practice.* St. Louis: Elsevier; 2016.

FIG. 1.14 Goals and interventions are developed and included in a patient's plan of care in collaboration with the patient, health care team members, and others involved in the patient's care. (From Bulechek G, Butcher H, Dochterman J, et al. *Nursing interventions classification [NIC].* 6th ed. St. Louis: Elsevier; 2013 and Moorhead S, Johnson M, Mass M, et al. *Nursing outcomes classification [NOC].* 5th ed. St. Louis: Elsevier; 2013).

involving direct or indirect nursing care. Direct care is provided by having personal contact with patients. It may require reassessment by the nurse, physical care such as assisting with a patient's activities of daily living or starting an IV line, informal counseling, or teaching. Indirect care is provided to patients by nurses through communication and collaboration with others involved in the patient's care, referrals to other health care providers or facilities, research, advocacy, or delegation. Some interventions are independent nursing actions within the nursing scope of practice such as repositioning a patient or providing emotional support, whereas others are dependent nursing actions requiring orders from the

Box 1.2 Resources for Planning Patient-Centered Care

Ackley B, Ladwig G. *Nursing diagnosis handbook: An evidence-based guide to planning care*. 11th ed. St. Louis: Elsevier; 2016.

Bulechek G, Butcher H, Dochterman J, Wagner C. *Nursing interventions classification (NIC)*. 6th ed. St. Louis: Elsevier; 2013.

Gulanick M, Myers J. *Nursing care plans: Diagnosis, interventions, and outcomes*. 8th ed. St. Louis: Elsevier; 2014.

Herdman T, Kamitsuru S. *Nursing diagnosis: Definitions and classification 2015-2017*. West Sussex, UK: Wiley Blackwell; 2014.

International Classification for Nursing Practice (ICNP®). (2015). Available at http://www.icn.ch/what-we-do/international-classification-for-nursing-practice-icnpr/.

Moorhead S, Johnson M, Maas M, Swanson E. *Nursing outcomes classification (NOC): Measurement of health outcomes*. 5th ed. St. Louis: Elsevier; 2013.

Swearingen P. *All-in-one nursing care planning resource: Medical-surgical, pediatric, maternity, and psychiatric-mental health*. 4th ed. St. Louis: Elsevier; 2016.

Evaluation

Goal met.
Continue plan of care.
Patient walking in hallway within 24 hours with R 20 and unlabored without supplement oxygen, P 88 and regular.

FIG. 1.15 Evaluation is patient focused and is the final step of the nursing process recorded on the Conceptual Care Map (CCM).

patient's primary care provider. In all cases, the patient's needs and best practice determine which interventions are included in the patient's plan of care.

The final area of the CCM requires the nurse to document: (1) the patient's status related to the attainment of goals or outcomes, (2) if the goal was met or not met, and (3) a determination as to whether the plan of care should be continued, discontinued, or revised to better address the patient's need. Similar to goal statements, evaluation is totally patient focused rather than nursing focused. Fig. 1.15 illustrates evaluation of the patient's goal attainment on the CCM and includes all three required aspects. The best evaluation statements begin with the patient as the subject.

The quality and effectiveness of a patient's plan of care is dependent on several factors. These include the accuracy and thoroughness of assessment data, effective communication and collaboration with the patient and various members of the health care team, and strong critical thinking and clinical decision-making skills of the nurse. Combined with research, these factors are crucial in providing safe, cost-effective, patient-centered care.

REFERENCE

Yoost B, Crawford L. *Fundamentals of nursing: Active learning for collaborative practice*. St. Louis: Elsevier; 2016.

2

Assessment

Learning Outcomes

Comprehension of this chapter's content will provide students with the ability to:

LO 2.1   Identify strategies used to conduct patient assessment.

LO 2.2   Describe how to validate assessment data.

LO 2.3   Document patient data for care plan development.

Assessment data must be collected, validated, and organized by the nurse before developing a patient-centered, research-based plan of care. Initial assessment information provides a baseline for comparison of future findings. Data collection continues during each patient-nurse encounter, providing additional information from which the nurse can identify specific patient problems, goals, and interventions. The process of collecting and organizing patient information requires that the nurse incorporates several strategies to ensure a thorough approach to assessment.

Strategies for Patient Assessment   LO 2.1

Five basic strategies are used by the nurse to gain insight into a patient's condition. These include observing the patient and situation, reviewing the patient's health record, interviewing the patient, conducting a health history, and completing a physical examination. The process of assessment begins when the nurse reads a patient's health record or observes the patient for the first time.

Observation

Observation of a patient often reveals significant information about the patient's emotional state, affect, personal hygiene, pride in appearance, and physical impairment, such as a limp (Fig. 2.1). The skill of observation improves throughout a student's or nurse's practice as knowledge of various physical and emotional conditions increases. Using the senses of sight, hearing, and smell during the observation phase of assessment helps the nurse to obtain vital patient data. Observed findings provide the nurse with basic information to explore more fully during a review of health records and the patient interview.

Health Record Review

Before initiating a patient interview, the nurse should review the patient's health records to become familiar with information recorded previously by other health care professionals. Prior lab and diagnostic test results as well as medication and health history information provide insight into the patient's overall wellness. For instance, if the patient's health record indicates no prior illness, and includes only annual physical exam findings, the nurse's approach to assessing the patient will be vastly different than if the patient has an extensive health record revealing multiple injuries or illnesses for which the person has been treated.

Reviewing health record information before initiating significant patient contact saves time and communicates concern to the patient. If a patient is asked to repeat information that is already documented, it may cause the patient to become frustrated and diminish the level of initial trust within the nurse-patient relationship. Documented information from a patient's health record should be used by the nurse as a basis on which to ask further questions of clarification during the interview process.

Patient Interview

The patient interview is a formal, structured discussion in which the nurse questions the patient to obtain demographic information, data about current health concerns, and medical and surgical histories. During the assessment process, it is essential for the nurse to gather information regarding developmental, cultural, ethnic, and spiritual factors that may affect the patient. These factors can significantly influence patient outcomes and must be considered when developing a patient-centered plan of care.

Patients who feel accepted and relaxed in the health care environment are more likely to disclose vital information to the nurse during the interview and physical examination. The patient interview consists of three phases: orientation (or introductory), working, and termination. Each phase contributes to the development of trust and engagement between the nurse and the patient. During the orientation phase, the nurse establishes the name that the patient wants to be called, provides a personal introduction, and states the purpose of the interview. Timing and location of the interview are important to provide for the patient's comfort and privacy. It is best for the nurse to be seated or stand at eye level with the patient and observe for nonverbal behaviors that provide insight into the patient's condition (Fig. 2.2).

During the working phase of the interview, the nurse must stay focused on the purpose of the interaction. The nurse needs to individualize the process on the basis of the health of the patient and concerns that emerge during the course of the interview. Active, engaged listening is imperative during this process. The nurse must stay alert to what the patient says and how information is presented. Sometimes, how the patient shares information is more important than what the patient says. Box 2.1 highlights some nurse behaviors that research has identified as important to patient satisfaction and safety. Educational needs are assessed during the patient interview. The nurse should document gaps in patient knowledge and areas in which

clarification of disease processes or treatment would be beneficial. Knowing a patient's level of education and professional background is often helpful in designing appropriate patient teaching strategies.

A variety of communication techniques can be incorporated into the interview process. Open-ended questions encourage narrative responses from patients. Closed-ended, focused, and direct questions elicit specific information, such as the exact location of a patient's pain. It is appropriate to use direct questions to gather data about a patient's health history, or during the review of body systems, when a yes or no answer is adequate. Direct questions can be expanded on with open-ended questions if more

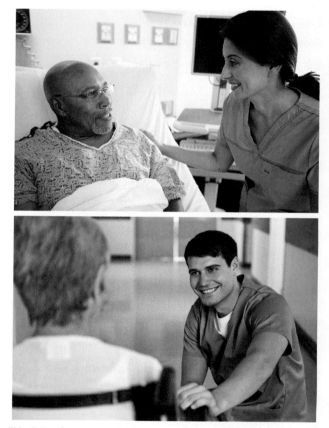

FIG. 2.2 Communicating with patients at eye level enhances the ability of the nurse to observe nonverbal behaviors and demonstrates patient respect.

Box 2.1 Nursing Behaviors During the Interview

Research has identified several nursing behaviors that contribute to patient satisfaction and safety and should be implemented during the interview process:
- Summarizing and repeating information.
- Explaining medical terminology.
- Providing a room with adequate privacy.
- Involving family and friends as requested by the patient.

From Uphoff E, Wennekes L, Punt CJ, et al. Development of generic quality indicators for patient-centered cancer care by using a RAND Modified Delphi Method. *Cancer Nurs.* 2012;35(1):29-37.

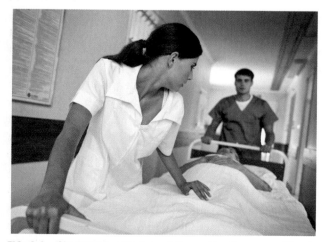

FIG. 2.1 Observing a patient carefully provides the nurse with valuable baseline assessment data.

extensive information is needed. Chapter 3 provides additional information on therapeutic communication techniques that are helpful to incorporate during the patient interview. The termination phase of the interview takes place after the nurse conducts an in-depth health history including a review of systems.

Health History

An in-depth health history includes all pertinent information that can guide the development of a patient-centered plan of care. The health history includes demographic data, which is collected during the orientation phase of the interview; a patient's chief complaint, or reason for seeking health care; history of current illness; allergies; medications; adverse reactions to medications; medical history; family and social history; and health promotion practices (Table 2.1). All findings should be documented in chronological order to provide a clear picture of the patient's health care concerns and their progression across time.

Review of Systems

A review of systems, which is conducted by asking the patient questions pertaining to each body system, completes the health history. During the review of systems, the nurse collects subjective, patient-reported data. Questions asked during the review of systems usually are brief and enquire about the normal function of each area. Any deviation from normal triggers more directive questions by the nurse to provide greater clarity of the patient's condition, and affects the physical assessment.

Physical Examination

Following the patient interview, health history, and review of systems, the nurse begins the physical exam. During the physical assessment, the nurse collects objective data. If diagnostic tests, such as blood tests or x-rays, were ordered before the patient was seen, the results are reviewed by the nurse. Privacy for the patient is ensured, good lighting is established, and the equipment and instruments needed are gathered before the physical examination is started. Box 2.2 provides a list of equipment needed to conduct a complete physical assessment. Vital signs are taken and recorded at the beginning of the physical examination. The assessment techniques of inspection, palpation, percussion, and auscultation are performed one at a time in this order for each body system except during assessment of the abdomen. During abdominal assessment, auscultation precedes palpation and percussion.

Depending on the practice setting, the nurse will conduct one of three primary types of physical assessment. Each provides varying amounts of patient information based on the timing and situation of the nurse-patient interaction. An initial comprehensive or complete physical examination should be performed by a nurse when a patient is admitted to the hospital. It can be followed by clinical or focused assessments at the beginning of each shift or more often, depending on the patient's condition and the health care facility's policies and guidelines. Emergency assessments, including triage, are conducted in emergent situations to quickly assess the extent of patient injuries and determine care priorities. It is the responsibility of the nurse to determine if a patient's condition warrants more frequent or extensive assessment in any given situation. A patient's plan of care is evaluated and modified on the basis of the assessment findings collected during every type of assessment.

Data Validation   LO 2.2

Observing and listening carefully to patients elicits helpful and sometimes confusing data which the nurse must validate to determine its significance to the patient's condition. For instance, the nurse may notice that a patient's affect is flat, possibly indicating indifference or depression, or a patient may be limping, indicative of a new or earlier injury, or congenital condition. When a patient exhibits either physical or emotional deviations from what is expected, these cues are potential indications of a disease or disorder and require further investigation by the nurse to validate what is observed. Ideas of what may be the underlying cause of a patient's observed behavior cannot be assumed.

Data validation is critical to ensure that patient information is accurate. As patient information is collected, consistency between subjective (stated) data and objective (observed) data must be confirmed. Sometimes subjective data can be validated through vital sign assessment, or laboratory and diagnostic tests. For instance, if a patient's skin is flushed, taking the patient's temperature and monitoring for an increase in the patient's white blood cell (WBC) count can verify the reason for the patient's appearance (Fig. 2.3). Each time the nurse encounters a patient, family member, or care giver, additional data is collected that needs to be validated in the context of initial assessment information.

Sometimes the nurse will notice a subtle change in a patient's condition or a potentially troublesome family interaction that requires interpretation. When interpreting information, the nurse must be careful to avoid inaccurate inferences (assumptions) that may be based solely on the nurse's past experiences, generalizations, personal preferences, or outdated health care information. Interpreting data and making inferences that determine patient care must involve ongoing interaction with patients and others, which includes sensitivity to the patient's expectations, cultural and ethnic traditions, and values.

Table 2.1 Framework for Collecting Health History Data

Type of Data	Specific Information	Type of Data	Specific Information
Demographic data	Name Address Telephone numbers Age Birth date Birthplace Gender Marital status Race Cultural background or ethnic origin Spiritual or religious preference Educational level Occupation	Family history	Age and health status of living parents, grandparents, siblings, and children Age at death and cause of death of deceased immediate family members Genetic diseases or traits, familial diseases (e.g., cardiovascular disease, high blood pressure, stroke, blood disorders, cancer, diabetes, kidney disease, seizure disorders, drug or alcohol dependencies, mental illness)
Chief complaint or current illness	Reason for seeking care Onset of symptoms	Social history	Use of tobacco, alcohol, or recreational drugs Environmental exposures Animal exposures and pets Living arrangement Safety concerns (e.g., intimate-partner violence, emotional or physical abuse) Recent domestic or foreign travel
Allergies and sensitivities	Medication Food (e.g., peanuts, eggs) Environmental agents (e.g., latex, tape, detergents) Reaction to reported allergens (e.g., rash, breathing difficulty, nausea, vomiting) Contrast dye	Cultural and spiritual or religious traditions	Primary language Dietary restrictions Religion Values and beliefs related to health care
Medications, vitamins, and herbal supplements	Prescription Over-the-counter medications and herbal remedies Dosage, frequency, and reason for use	Activities of daily living (ADLs)	Nutrition (e.g., meal preparation, shopping, typical 24-hour dietary intake); recent changes in appetite Caffeine intake Self-care activities (e.g., bathing, dressing, grooming, ambulation) Physical living environment (e.g., steps, access to toileting or sleeping areas, indoor plumbing, carpet or rugs) Use of prosthetics or mobility devices Leisure and exercise activities Sleep patterns (e.g., hours per night, naps, sleep aids)
Immunizations	Childhood and adult immunizations Date of last tuberculin skin test Date of last vaccines (e.g., flu, pneumonia, shingles)		
Medical history	Childhood illnesses, accidents, and injuries Serious or chronic illnesses Hospitalizations, including obstetric history for female patients Date of occurrence and current treatment	Cognitive or emotional status	Cognitive functioning Personal strengths Self-esteem Support system (e.g., family, friend, support groups, professional counseling)
Surgical history	Type of surgery Date Problems with anesthesia Any complications		

From Yoost BL, Crawford LR. *Fundamentals of nursing: Active learning for collaborative practice.* St. Louis: Elsevier; 2016.

Accurate interpretation of patient data requires the nurse to understand disease processes, vital sign parameters, typical physical assessment findings, and normal values and outcomes for laboratory and diagnostic tests. The nurse must know typical signs and symptoms of disease processes and which laboratory and diagnostic test results should be monitored on the basis of a patient's condition and medical diagnosis. After the nurse has collected, reviewed, validated, and interpreted patient information as accurately as possible it is documented in the patient's health record.

Documentation for Care Plan Development   LO 2.3

Documenting patient information allows access by multiple members of the health care team, facilitates communication of essential data, and continuity of care. Electronic health records use a variety of methods for data organization and documentation. The first section of the Conceptual Care Map (CCM) mimics various forms used by hospitals and clinics for assessment data entry while providing a visual map of patient data (Fig. 2.4). Once patient data is recorded in the seven subsections of the assessment area of the CCM, the student or nurse can analyze relationships between or among two or more pieces of collected patient information. It is in synthesizing patient data that disease etiologies and rationales for various orders, treatments, and changes in status become clear.

After patient assessment data is organized and documented accurately, the nurse reviews best practices revealed through research and collaborates with members of the health care team to formulate a patient-centered plan of care. Guidelines for sharing patient medical information

---

Box 2.2 Equipment Used for Physical Examination

- Patient gown
- Scale
- Height assessment tool
- Sphygmomanometer with cuff
- Stethoscope with bell and diaphragm
- Thermometer
- Wrist watch
- Pulse oximeter
- Disposable pads and/or exam table paper
- Bath blanket or sheet
- Gloves
- Cotton applicators and/or cotton balls
- Eye chart
- Flashlight or penlight
- Otoscope and ophthalmoscope
- Tuning fork
- Tongue depressor
- Reflex hammer
- Tape measure or ruler
- Specimen containers, as needed

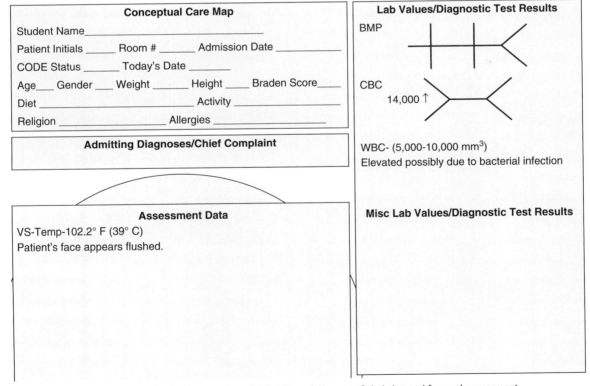

FIG. 2.3   Some subjective data can be validated through the use of vital sign and focused assessment, and/or laboratory or diagnostic testing.

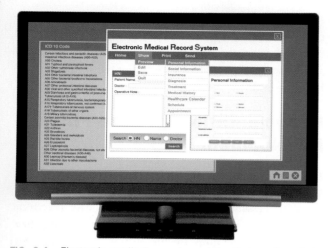

FIG. 2.4 Electronic medical records and the first section of the Conceptual Care Map require nurses and students to record similar patient data.

Nurses who are conducting patient physicals need to be aware of guidelines for sharing medical information:

- Patients are permitted to review their personal medical records.
  - This is one of many reasons that documentation should always be factual and nonjudgmental in nature.
  - Patients' review of their records should take place in the presence of the primary care provider to ensure accurate interpretation of the documentation.
- Family members may review the patient's medical records only with the written consent of the patient.
- Primary care providers and nurses are permitted to share patient medical information with members of the health care team involved in the patient's care without additional consent.
- Health care facilities require that patients sign a release form when requesting copies of their medical records or diagnostic test records.
- Nurses must respect the right of patients to know with whom their medical information can be legally shared.

From U.S. Department of Health and Human Services. Retrieved from www.hhs.gov/ocr/privacy/hipaa/understanding/consumers/index.html.

obtained during the assessment process are followed to ensure patient privacy and maintain professional ethical and legal standards of practice (Box 2.3).

As additional patient data becomes available, it is documented, trends are noted, and the nurse advocates for needed treatments or referrals to assist the patient to achieve established goals. Throughout care, assessment continues every second, minute, hour, or day, depending on the severity of the patient's condition. Assessment never stops. Therefore, documentation of findings is ongoing, impacting the patient's plan of care. Care plans evolve as patient needs change. Communication with the patient, family members, care givers, and each member of the health care team is critical to determining acceptable treatment options and for achieving the best possible patient outcomes.

CHAPTER 3

Communication

Learning Outcomes

Comprehension of this chapter's content will provide students with the ability to:

LO 3.1 Discuss various modes of communication.
LO 3.2 Describe communication components necessary for professional nursing practice.
LO 3.3 Differentiate between therapeutic and nontherapeutic communication techniques.
LO 3.4 Identify handoff communication strategies to improve patient safety.

Communication is the key to human relationships and patient safety. It requires effort and attention to detail. Communication impacts all aspects of nursing care from initial assessment to patient discharge and beyond. In 60% of sentinel health care events (resulting in unexpected death or permanent loss of function) that occurred between January 2013 and September 2015, communication breakdown was identified as one of the top three causes (The Joint Commission, 2015). To be viewed as competent, a nurse's communication skills must be professional and credible. Understanding the various modes in which individuals communicate, the skills of therapeutic communication, and the strategies for thorough handoffs can greatly enhance the ability of a nurse to effectively care for patients and their families.

Modes of Communication
LO 3.1

Many methods are used to convey information, however there are only two basic modes of communication: verbal and nonverbal. Verbal communication may be spoken, written, or electronic. Nonverbal communication is revealed in the form of body language such as gestures, eye contact, and voice inflection. Both basic modes of communication are critical to nursing practice. To effectively assess patients, nurses must skillfully observe and listen, requiring attention to both nonverbal and verbal communication. Establishing the true meaning of communication requires the nurse to watch for congruency between that which is being shared verbally and nonverbal cues.

Nonverbal Communication

Nonverbal communication is wordless transmission of information. A majority of communication is nonverbal, and it is the more accurate mode of conveying information. Realizing the frequency and value of nonverbal communication helps the nurse to observe and assess patients more accurately. Nurses who perceive the potential effect of their own nonverbal behavior will communicate more professionally and consistently when interacting with others. Nonverbal communication is totally absent in written and electronic communication, sometimes making it difficult to interpret. When communication lacks nonverbal cues, the nurse must verify its meaning to avoid making false assumptions.

Body Language

Body language is conveyed in many ways. Posture, stance, gait, facial expressions, eye movements, touch, gestures, and symbolic expressions influencing personal appearance, such as jewelry and make-up, generally communicate a person's thoughts more accurately than simple verbal interactions. The nurse needs to observe patients and family members for nonverbal cues while interviewing or completing assessments (Fig. 3.1). Cultural and ethnic differences, mental health issues, and physical and emotional states affect the way people communicate.

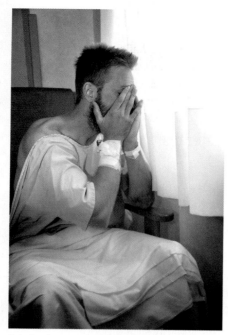

FIG. 3.1 A patient's nonverbal behavior may be an indication of pain or an emotion such as frustration, requiring further assessment by the nurse to validate its meaning.

Voice Inflection

Another significant form of nonverbal communication is voice inflection. Spoken words may be emphasized through tone, volume, and the rhythm or rate of speech. Nurses must actively listen to perceive the quality of speech used during interactions with others. Voice inflection provides insight into the significance of information being shared.

Verbal Communication

Verbal communication is shared as spoken, written, or electronic information. In most cases, nurses combine it with nonverbal cues obtained through observation and assessment to establish its full meaning and accuracy. Spoken words may be communicated face to face, in a group setting, or through devices such as phones or intercoms. The setting in which communication takes place greatly influences what is or what can be shared. The context and content of verbal communication must be closely monitored by the nurse to avoid misinterpretation or errors in patient care.

Written communication, although effective in providing details and legal documentation, lacks the nuances that voice inflection and interactive conversation can provide. The meaning of written communication is often enhanced through discussion. Oral reports or grand rounds typically highlight the urgency of patient needs more than written documentation.

Electronic communication in the form of information referencing, e-mail, social networking, and blogging can quickly contribute to a person's knowledge, providing patients and health care professionals with vital information. However, the potential for miscommunication exists, in part because nonverbal cues are not apparent. When communicating verbally by electronic media, patients and nurses must take time to validate and verify shared information because misunderstandings can occur if feedback is inadequate.

Communication Components Necessary for Nursing Practice   LO 3.2

Respect, assertiveness, collaboration, delegation, and advocacy are critical components of professional nursing communication that facilitate positive patient outcomes. Respecting patients and advocating on their behalf builds trust and conveys caring. Collaborating and delegating assertively with health care team members creates a positive work environment focused on patient needs.

Respect

Respect for patients and their families is conveyed by nurses verbally and nonverbally. Asking a patient's name preference during initial contact demonstrates respect and establishes the foundation for a trusting nurse–patient relationship. Ensuring privacy, providing necessary health care information, and fostering autonomy in decision making are nursing actions that further strengthen the relationship. Controlling facial expressions and body language during challenging interactions with patients and health care team members is essential to consistently demonstrate respect.

Assertiveness

Assertiveness is the ability to express ideas and concerns clearly while respecting the thoughts of others. Assertive nurses communicate with patients, families, and other members of the health care team regularly and without hesitation. Assertive communication by nurses demonstrates confidence and elicits respect from patients and colleagues. Overly assertive nurses may be perceived as aggressive if they do not respect the rights and opinions of others. Nurses who communicate aggressively tend to receive negative or defensive responses from patients, family members, and health care team members.

Collaboration

Collaboration with other health care professionals is a key factor in communicating necessary health care information and providing comprehensive patient care. Most patients require the collaboration of many different health

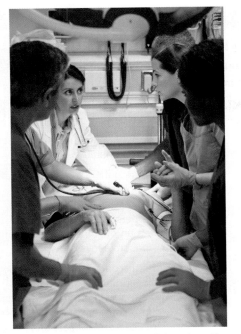

FIG. 3.2 Effective communication and collaboration with members of the health care team is essential to patient safety.

care professionals during hospitalization or outpatient treatment, and the nurse is often the coordinator of this team (Fig. 3.2). Physicians, nurse practitioners, laboratory technicians, social workers, and respiratory, physical, occupational, and speech therapists, along with unlicensed assistive personnel, may share responsibility for patient care. The nurse must contact key health care professionals in an expedient manner and with respect and recognition of time and resource limitations. Ongoing communication with the patient about the status of the health care team collaboration is essential to allay unnecessary anxiety associated with not knowing what is happening. Chapter 4 provides further information on the importance of collaboration in health care.

Delegation

Delegation is a multifaceted responsibility of the registered nurse. When communicating during delegation, nurses must show collegiality and respect for all members of the health care team. It is important to call other health care team members by their preferred names. Accuracy while communicating ensures positive patient outcomes. Receiving feedback from the person to whom care is delegated is required by law and provides an opportunity for clarity, which ensures greater accuracy.

Communicating therapeutically with colleagues during the delegation process shows respect and recognizes the many stressors with which all members of the health care team cope while providing patient care. Offers of support and encouragement help convey empathy and promote teamwork.

Advocacy

Patient advocacy is a hallmark of professional nursing. Advocacy involves defending the rights of others, especially those who are vulnerable or unable to make decisions independently. To be an effective advocate for patients, the nurse must be knowledgeable, organized, and able to communicate in a caring manner. Nurses who communicate therapeutically and assertively are better able to advocate for their patients.

Therapeutic and Nontherapeutic Communication LO 3.3

There is a significant difference between casual, social interaction, and therapeutic communication (i.e., beneficial, positive interaction). The primary focus of therapeutic communication between a patient and nurse is the patient. Nurses engaged in therapeutic conversations set their own opinions and judgments aside to listen more fully to their patients. Through various techniques, such as active listening, open posture, and reflection, nurses encourage patients to explore personal concerns. Patients often respond with open, honest sharing to nurses who are accepting of alternative ideas and empathetic to the circumstances of others. Nurses need to value the important role of therapeutic and open dialogue in the healing process.

Therapeutic Communication

The use of therapeutic communication techniques enhances nurse–patient relationships and helps to achieve positive outcomes. Consistent use demonstrates empathy and concern for patients. Various techniques greatly assist the nurse in gathering, verifying, and validating assessment data. Table 3.1 provides examples and rationales for verbal therapeutic communication techniques that nurses should practice while providing care within all settings. Table 3.2 highlights examples and rationales for some essential nonverbal therapeutic techniques that nurses should implement when communicating with patients.

Nontherapeutic Communication

Nontherapeutic communication can be hurtful and potentially damaging to nurse–patient interaction. Changing the subject (e.g., in response to a patient who expresses a desire to talk about a concern that makes the nurse uncomfortable) or sharing personal opinions limits conversation between the nurse and the patient and discourages open conversation on sensitive topics. Many aspects of social conversation should be avoided when interacting with patients. Most are considered nontherapeutic and tend to shift the conversational focus away from the patient's

Table 3.1 Verbal Techniques for Initiating and Encouraging Communication

Technique	Examples	Rationale
Offering self	"I'll sit with you for a while." "I'll stay with you until your family member arrives."	• Demonstrates compassion and concern for the patient • Establishes a caring relationship
Calling the patient by name	"Good morning, Mr. Trimble." "Hi, Ms. Martin. How are you feeling this evening?"	• Conveys that the nurse sees the patient as an individual • Shows respect and helps to establish a caring relationship
Sharing observations	"You look tense." "You seem frustrated." "You are smiling."	• Raises the patient's awareness of his or her nonverbal behavior • Allows the patient to validate the nurse's perceptions • Provides an opening for the patient to share possible joys or concerns
Giving information	"It is time for your bath." "My name is Pam, and I will be the RN taking care of you until 7 p.m." "Your surgery is scheduled for 10:30 a.m. tomorrow."	• Informs the patient of facts needed in a specific situation • Provides a means to build trust and develop a knowledge base on which patients can make decisions
Using open-ended questions or comments	"What are some of your biggest concerns?" "Tell me more about your general health status." "Share some of the feelings you experienced after your heart attack."	• Gives the patient the opportunity to share freely on a subject • Avoids interjection of feelings or assumptions by the nurse • Provides for patient elaboration on important topics when the nurse wants to collect a breadth of information
Using focused questions or comments	"Point to exactly where your pain is radiating." "When did you start experiencing shortness of breath?" "How has your family responded to your being hospitalized?" "What is your greatest fear?" "Where were you when the symptoms started?" "Tell me where you live."	• Encourages the patient to share specific data necessary for completing a thorough assessment • Asks the patient to provide details regarding various concerns • Focuses on the immediate needs of the patient
Providing general leads	"And then?" "Go on." "Tell me more."	• Encourages the patient to keep talking • Demonstrates the nurse's interest in the patient's concerns
Conveying acceptance	"Yes." Nodding. "I follow what you are saying." "Uh huh."	• Acknowledges the importance of the patient's thoughts, feelings, and concerns
Using humor	"You are really walking well this morning. I'm going to have to run to catch up!"	• Provides encouragement • May lighten heavy moments of discussion • Used properly, allows a patient to focus on positive progress or better times and does not change the subject of a conversation
Verbalizing the implied	Patient: "I can't talk to anyone about this." Nurse: "Do you feel that others won't understand?"	• Encourages a patient to elaborate on a topic of concern • Provides an opportunity for the patient to articulate more clearly a complicated topic or feeling that could be easily misunderstood
Paraphrasing or restating communication content	Patient: "I couldn't sleep last night." Nurse: "You had trouble sleeping last night?"	• Encourages patients to describe situations more fully • Demonstrates that the nurse is listening
Reflecting feelings or emotions	"You were angry when your surgery was delayed?" "You seem excited about going home today."	• Focuses on the patient's identified feelings based on verbal or nonverbal cues

Table 3.1 Verbal Techniques for Initiating and Encouraging Communication—cont'd

Technique	Examples	Rationale
Seeking clarification	"I don't quite follow what you are saying." "What do you mean by your last statement?"	• Encourages the patient to expand on a topic that may be confusing or that seems contradictory
Summarizing	"There are three things you are upset about: your family being too busy, your diet, and being in the hospital too long."	• Reduces the interaction to three or four points identified by the nurse as being significant • Allows the patient to agree or add additional concerns
Validating	"Did I understand you correctly that...?"	• Allows clarification of ideas that the nurse may have interpreted differently than intended by the patient

From Yoost BL, Crawford LR. *Fundamentals of nursing: Active learning for collaborative practice.* St. Louis: Elsevier; 2016.

Table 3.2 Nonverbal Techniques for Facilitating Communication

Technique	Examples	Rationale
Active listening	• Maintaining intermittent eye contact • Matching eye levels • Attentive posturing • Facing the patient • Leaning toward the person who is speaking • Avoiding distracting body movement	• Conveys interest in the patient's needs, concerns, or problems • Provides the patient with undivided attention • Sends a clear message of concern and interest
Silence	• Being present with a person without verbal communication	• Provides the patient time to think or reflect • Communicates concern when there is really nothing adequate to say in difficult or challenging situations
Therapeutic touch	• Holding the hand of a patient • Providing a backrub • Touching a patient's arm lightly • Shaking hands with a patient in isolation	• Conveys empathy • Provides emotional support, encouragement, and personal attention • Relaxes the patient

From Yoost BL, Crawford LR. *Fundamentals of nursing: Active learning for collaborative practice.* St. Louis: Elsevier; 2016.

concerns. Nurses engaging in nontherapeutic social conversation tend to be labeled by patients as uncaring and self-absorbed. Table 3.3 provides examples of nontherapeutic communication that should be avoided. Avoiding nontherapeutic communication requires practice and experience. Intentionally incorporating as many therapeutic communication strategies as possible into conversations helps a nurse better meet patients' needs.

Handoff Communication   LO 3.4

The real-time process of passing patient-specific information from one caregiver to another or among health care team members to ensure continuity of care and patient safety is commonly referred to as a *handoff.* The Joint Commission (2015) determined that handoff communication was the number one root cause of transfer-related sentinel events between January 2004 and September 2015. Handoffs can be oral, as in a face-to-face meeting or telephone communication, or they can be written, documented in the electronic health record (EHR), or voice recorded (i.e., discharge summary). The information exchange can take place between providers, between shifts, and at the time of unit transfer or discharge referral.

Transitioning patients from one type of care to another (e.g., acute care to long-term care, intensive care unit to medical-surgical unit) involves risks because of a lack of uniformity in the handoff process and inadequate training on how to communicate during the transfer of care. When complete and accurate information is not shared during a handoff report, patients may not get needed care, proper medications, or recommended therapies. It is critically important that nurses pay attention to detail during the handoff procedure.

Handoffs include accurate and timely information about the care, treatment (i.e., medication reconciliation, physical therapy), and services (i.e., language interpretation, ambulation equipment) provided to a patient,

Table 3.3 Nontherapeutic Communication

Action	Examples	Rationale
Asking "why" questions	"Why did you do that?" "Why are you feeling that way?" "Why do you continue to smoke when you know it is unhealthy?"	• Implies criticism • May make the patient defensive • Tends to limit conversation • Requires justification of actions • Focuses on a problem rather than a possible solution
Using closed-ended questions or comments	"Do you feel better today?" "Did you sleep well last night?" "Have you made a decision about radiation yet?" "Are you ready to take your bath?" "Will you let me give you your medicine now?"	• Results in short, one-word, yes or no responses • Limits elaboration or discussion of a topic • Allows patient to refuse important care • Differs from focused questions that direct an interview
Changing the subject	Patient: "I'm having a difficult time talking with my daughter." Nurse: "Do you have grandchildren?" Patient: "I just want to die." Nurse: "Did you sleep well last night?"	• Avoids exploration of the topic raised by the patient • Demonstrates the nurse's discomfort with the topic introduced by the patient
Giving false reassurance	"Everything will be okay." "Surgery is nothing to be concerned about." "Don't worry; everything will be fine."	• Discounts the patient's feelings • Cuts off conversation about legitimate concerns of the patient • Demonstrates a need by the nurse to "fix" something that the patient just wants to discuss
Giving advice	"If it were me, I would…" "You should really exercise more." "You should absolutely have chemotherapy to treat your breast cancer if you expect to live." "Of course you should tell your co-workers that you've been diagnosed with cancer."	• Discourages the patient from finding an appropriate solution to a personal problem • Tends to limit the patient's ability to explore alternative solutions to issues that need to be faced • Implies a lack of confidence in the patient to make a healthy decision • Removes the decision-making authority from the patient
Giving stereotypical or generalized responses	"It's for your own good." "Keep your chin up." "Don't cry over spilt milk." "You will be home before long."	• Discounts patient feelings or opinions • Limits further conversation on a topic • May be perceived as judgmental
Showing approval or disapproval	"That's good." "You have no reason to be crying."	• Limits reflection by patients • Stops further discussion on patient decisions or actions • Implies a need for patients to have the nurse's support and approval
Showing agreement or disagreement	"That's right." "I disagree with what you just said."	• Discontinues patient reflection on an introduced topic • Implies a lack of value for the thoughts, feelings, or concerns of patients
Engaging in excessive self-disclosure or comparing the experiences of others	"I had the same type of cancer 2 years ago." "I have several family members who drink too much, too." "I go to that restaurant every Friday for fish."	• Implies that experiences related to a disease process are similar for all patients • Takes the focus away from the patient • Limits further reflection or problem solving by the patient
Comparing patient experiences	"The lady in room 250 just had this surgery last week and did just fine." "My uncle had this type of inflammatory bowel disease and ended up having to have a colostomy."	• Removes the focus of conversation from the patient • Invalidates each individual patient experience as being unique and important • Breaches confidentiality

Table 3.3 Nontherapeutic Communication—cont'd

Action	Examples	Rationale
Using personal terms of endearment	"Honey." "Sweetie, it is time to take your medicine." "Sport, how about if you show me how well you can walk across the room?"	• Demonstrates disrespect for the individual • Diminishes the dignity of a unique patient • May indicate that the nurse did not take the time or care enough to learn or remember the patient's name
Being defensive	"The nurses here work very hard." "Your doctor is extremely busy." "This is the best hospital in the area." "You won't get any better care anywhere else."	• Moves the focus from the patient • Discounts the patient's feelings and thoughts on a subject • Limits further conversation on a topic of patient concern

From Yoost BL, Crawford LR. *Fundamentals of nursing: Active learning for collaborative practice.* St. Louis: Elsevier; 2016.

Table 3.4 Situation, Background, Assessment, and Recommendation Communication Tool

Element	Action
Situation	Briefly describe the current concern or problem.
Background	Identify the circumstances or contributing factors of the current situation.
Assessment	Share pertinent data findings and critical analysis of the situation.
Recommendation	Suggest interventions based on best practice and sound clinical reasoning.

From Institute for Healthcare Improvement: *SBAR Toolkit*, 2014. Developed by Kaiser Permanente (Oakland, CA). www.ihi.org/resources/Pages/Tools/sbartoolkit.aspx.

addressing the patient's current condition and anticipated changes. They transfer authority and responsibility for care, which are legal concerns for nurses. Patient safety issues are heightened when information is transferred during intra-hospital transport. An ineffective handoff may lead to wrong treatments, wrong medications, or other life-threatening events, increasing the length of stay and causing patient injury or death. Improvement in the handoff process can increase patient safety and promote positive patient outcomes.

Standardized Handoff Procedures

Implementing a standardized process for handoffs is the best way to avoid errors. In some cases, this includes bedside shift reports with incoming staff, outgoing staff, and the patient. In other situations, handoffs are conducted during interdisciplinary care conferences and grand rounds. Regardless of the environment, standardizing handoff procedures have become a requirement in health care to provide for greater patient safety.

Situation, Background, Assessment, and Recommendation Model

A communication format specifically suggested for use in handoff interactions is SBAR (situation, background, assessment, and recommendation), a situation-briefing tool used by the U.S. Navy and adapted for health care (Table 3.4). The SBAR model, not unlike the nursing process, begins with the active situation, the related background, the assessment of the problem, and a recommendation for a solution. Using SBAR to organize and present handoff patient information standardizes the method by which information is shared, making it less likely that key data is missed. Standardized practices are endorsed by the Quality and Safety Education for Nurses Institute (QSEN), National Academy of Medicine (formerly the Institute of Medicine [IOM]), and others as a method of promoting patient safety and improving the quality of care.

Research continues to be conducted in a variety of health care settings to try to determine the best method of standardized handoff communication. At this time, SBAR is the most commonly used tool for nursing change-of-shift and transfer report. However, other methods are in use at some health care institutions. Regardless of the tool used by a health care facility, the focus for nurses and all interdisciplinary health care team members must always be patient safety and continuity of care.

REFERENCE

The Joint Commission. *Sentinel event data, 2004-3Q*; 2015. Available at: www.jointcommission.org/assets/1/18/Root_Causes_Event_Type_2004-3Q_2015.pdf.

CHAPTER

4

Collaboration

Learning Outcomes

Comprehension of this chapter's content will provide students with the ability to:

LO 4.1   Describe interprofessional collaboration in health care.

LO 4.2   Explain unique collaboration and delegation responsibilities of the nurse when working with licensed and unlicensed personnel.

LO 4.3   Discuss how collaboration enhances patient safety and positive patient outcomes.

Collaboration is the process by which two or more people work together toward a common goal. In health care, collaboration includes interaction among a wide variety of licensed and unlicensed personnel. Members of the interdisciplinary health care team vary depending on patient needs. Some of the participants who collaborate to provide care include but are not limited to:

- primary care providers (PCPs)
- medical specialist physicians
- surgical specialist physicians
- registered nurses (RNs)
- counselors
- dietitians
- social workers
- unlicensed assistive personnel (UAP)
- laboratory technicians
- pharmacists
- spiritual advisors (clergy, rabbis, imams, etc.)
- licensed practical/vocational nurses (LPNs/LVNs)
- speech pathologists and audiologists
- respiratory, physical, and occupational therapists

Requesting input from other members of the interdisciplinary health care team enhances a nurse's ability to meet the patient's needs. Each professional brings a different perspective and unique expertise that is valued.

Interprofessional Collaboration in Health Care   LO 4.1

Collaboration among health care professionals is essential to safe and effective patient care. The characteristics necessary for collaboration in health care are described in Box 4.1. The nurse's role includes coordinating patient care, making sure all patient care orders are carried out and goals are met, and communicating with the entire health care team. Chapter 3 provides additional information about communication among the health care team.

The Quality and Safety Education for Nurses (QSEN) initiative, funded by the Robert Wood Johnson Foundation

---

Box 4.1 Collaboration

Characteristics of collaboration among health care professionals include:
- Clinical competence and accountability
- Common purpose
- Interpersonal competence and effective communication
- Trust and mutual respect
- Recognition and valuation of diverse complementary knowledge and skills
- Humor

From Yoost BL, Crawford LR. *Fundamentals of nursing: Active learning for collaborative practice.* St. Louis: Elsevier; 2016.

Table 4.1 Teamwork and Collaboration

Definition: Function effectively within nursing and interprofessional teams, fostering open communication, mutual respect, and shared decision-making to achieve quality patient care.

KNOWLEDGE	SKILLS	ATTITUDES
Describe own strengths, limitations, and values in functioning as a member of a team	Demonstrate awareness of own strengths and limitations as a team member Initiate plan for self-development as a team member Act with integrity, consistency, and respect for differing views	Acknowledge own potential to contribute to effective team functioning Appreciate importance of intra- and interprofessional collaboration
Describe scopes of practice and roles of health care team members Describe strategies for identifying and managing overlaps in team member roles and accountabilities Recognize contributions of other individuals and groups in helping patient/family achieve health goals	Function competently within own scope of practice as a member of the health care team Assume role of team member or leader based on the situation Initiate requests for help when appropriate to situation Clarify roles and accountabilities under conditions of potential overlap in team-member functioning Integrate the contributions of others who play a role in helping patient/family achieve health goals	Value the perspectives and expertise of all health team members Respect the centrality of the patient/family as core members of any health care team Respect the unique attributes that members bring to a team, including variations in professional orientations and accountabilities
Analyze differences in communication style preferences among patients and families, nurses and other members of the health team Describe impact of own communication style on others Discuss effective strategies for communicating and resolving conflict	Communicate with team members, adapting own style of communicating to needs of the team and situation Demonstrate commitment to team goals Solicit input from other team members to improve individual, as well as team performance Initiate actions to resolve conflict	Value teamwork and the relationships upon which it is based Value different styles of communication used by patients, families, and health care providers Contribute to resolution of conflict and disagreement
Describe examples of the impact of team functioning on safety and quality of care Explain how authority gradients influence teamwork and patient safety	Follow communication practices that minimize risks associated with handoffs among providers and across transitions in care Assert own position/perspective in discussions about patient care Choose communication styles that diminish the risks associated with authority gradients among team members	Appreciate the risks associated with handoffs among providers and across transitions in care
Identify system barriers and facilitators of effective team functioning Examine strategies for improving systems to support team functioning	Participate in designing systems that support effective teamwork	Value the influence of system solutions in achieving effective team functioning

From Cronenwett L, Sherwood G, Barnsteiner J, et al. Quality and safety education for nurses. *Nurs Outlook*. 2007;55(3):122-131.

includes six competencies for nursing. One of the six competencies is *teamwork and collaboration*, which shows the significance of interdisciplinary teams working together. Knowledge, skills, and attitudes for each competency were developed for use in prelicensure and graduate nursing education. Table 4.1 outlines the knowledge, skills, and attitudes for the *teamwork and collaboration* competency for prelicensure nursing students (Cronenwett et al, 2007).

Different groups of professionals collaborate in the care of a patient depending on the setting and the patient's status. In the intensive care unit (ICU), registered nurses, intensivists, respiratory therapists, laboratory technicians, and physical therapists may collaborate to provide the urgent care needed in that setting. For a hospice patient, the team may include a primary care provider (PCP), hospice physician, hospice registered nurse (RN), spiritual leader, home health aide, social worker, and counselor (Fig. 4.1). After the nurse assesses a patient (see Chapter 2 for more information about assessment) and formulates a plan of care, others from the health care team may need to be

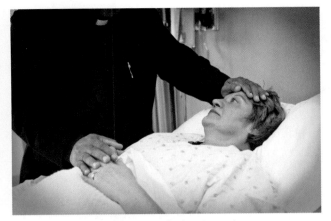

FIG. 4.1 A priest at the bedside of a hospice patient.

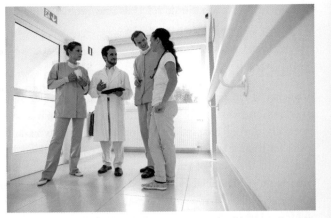

FIG. 4.2 Members of the health care team communicate and contribute unique perspectives.

consulted to help carry out the interventions necessary to attain patient goals.

Collaborative Interventions

Some patient interventions are implemented independently by the nurse, some are dependent on care provider orders, and others are collaborative. Collaborative interventions require the expertise of a few or many of the health care team members. They include activities such as physical therapy, hospice care, personal care, and spiritual counseling. Collaborative interventions necessitate consultation with other health care professionals or referral to specialists or agencies for assistance. Educational backgrounds and practice guidelines vary for each health care professional (Box 4.2). Examples of collaboration with some health care professionals are listed below. Nurses may collaborate with a(n):

• Registered dietitian when providing nutritional support while addressing medical or surgical conditions such as hypertension, dysphagia, or diabetes
• Physical therapist for assessment of the patient's mobility or crutch stability
• Occupational therapist for evaluation of the patient's activities of daily living (ADL)
• Speech therapist for assessment of a patient's ability to swallow or speech deficits
• Social worker to determine home care needs or hospitalization coverage

Interdisciplinary health care providers and patients need to communicate, and consider the unique perspective that each contributes (Fig. 4.2). This collaborative approach can better address the multiple factors that influence the health of patients. Individual providers cannot do this alone (Sullivan et al, 2015).

Referrals

Referrals in health care involve requesting that another member of the interdisciplinary health care team see a patient for a consultation or other services. In some cases, a PCP may refer a patient to a medical or surgical specialist for further assessment, testing, or treatment. Referral information provided by a specialist can provide the nurse and PCP with data for a more structured plan of care to address specific patient concerns.

Referrals for specialized services can support and protect patients. Nurses are often instrumental in initiating these types of referrals. For instance, if a patient is experiencing extreme anxiety during chemotherapy treatments, the nurse may set up a referral with the music therapist to assist the patient with relaxation. Nurses initiate referrals for specific dietary requests and adaptive care devices, depending on the patient's unique circumstances. In collaboration with a social worker, a nurse may refer discharged patients to community agencies that provide home care or other services suitable for the patient's situation. Some referrals may require the order of a physician or an advanced practice nurse.

Advocacy

Advocacy is the act of supporting a cause or recommending an action on behalf of others. Nurses are patient advocates especially during hospitalization, or when patients cannot speak for themselves. Even when nurses disagree philosophically with the plan of care, they are expected to focus on what is most beneficial for their patients. For example, the nurse may believe that a patient should undergo chemotherapy for colon cancer, whereas the patient's plan of care calls for placement in hospice care. The nurse needs to support the patient's desire and implement the care plan accordingly.

Advocacy is an important aspect of collaboration and coordination of patient care. Frequently, nurses must contact various referral agencies and network with several health care professionals to meet patient needs. The process of advocacy requires nurses to focus on the patient's needs and what interventions are of the greatest benefit.

Unique Collaboration and Delegation Responsibilities
LO 4.2

Nurses play a unique role within the interdisciplinary health care team. They are often coordinators of care, interacting with both licensed (physicians, social workers, licensed practical nurses/licensed vocation nurses [LPNs/LVNs]) and unlicensed ancillary personnel such as unlicensed assistive personnel (UAP), housekeepers, unit secretaries, janitors, and maintenance staff. Some of these individuals are involved in direct (hands-on) patient care, whereas others are not. Each member's role is recognized as an integral part of the team.

Collaboration with Ancillary Personnel

Although tasks are not specifically delegated by the RN to some ancillary workers, their role in a patient's recovery is valued. Often the nurse will interact with ancillary staff to improve the patient's experience and care in the hospital or long-term care setting. Examples of ancillary staff members assisting in the care and safety of patients include:
- Frequent cleaning of patient's rooms and disinfection of rooms by the housekeeping staff between patients to help prevent infection
- Repair of equipment such as intravenous (IV) pumps by the maintenance staff so that nurses can safely use the equipment in patient care
- Proper removal of trash and medical waste by the janitorial staff

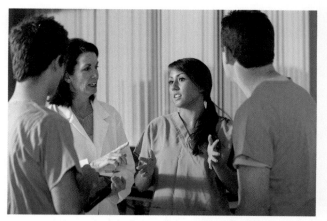

FIG. 4.3 The nurse delegates tasks to unlicensed assistive personnel and licensed practical nurses.

Box 4.3 Five Rights of Delegation

Collaboration among health care team members sometimes results in the nurse delegating some aspects of patient care to unlicensed assistive personnel. The National Council of State Boards of Nursing has provided the Five Rights of Delegation to support safe delegation of patient care:
1. *Right task:* Is this a task that can and should be delegated?
2. *Right circumstance:* Is this appropriate at this time with what is going on?
3. *Right person:* Does this person have the skills, scope of practice, understanding, and expertise to perform this task?
4. *Right direction or communication:* Has proper information about what tasks need to be completed been shared so that what needs to be done is clear?
5. *Right supervision or evaluation:* Has the nurse followed up to ensure that care was adequate to meet the needs of the patient?

From National Council of State Boards of Nursing. *The Five Rights of Delegation,* 1997. www.ncsbn.org/fiverights.pdf.

- Answering phones and performing clerical work by unit secretaries, tasks which are vital to the health care team's work.

All of these roles are crucial for excellence in patient care. It is a major responsibility of the nurse to make sure each member of the health care team is treated with respect and compassion.

Delegation

Nurses collaborate with certain members of the health care team through delegation. It is the process of entrusting or transferring the responsibility for certain tasks to some ancillary personnel, including UAP, and LPNs/LVNs (Fig. 4.3). Box 4.3 outlines the *Five Rights of Delegation.* The RN is responsible for knowing the scope of practice and capabilities of each health care team member as well as facility policy regarding what may be delegated. Some examples of patient care interventions that can and cannot be delegated to a UAP are listed in Box 4.4. Some interventions that may be delegated to the LPN/LVN include taking vital signs, administering oral medications, and obtaining finger stick blood glucose levels. The RN retains ultimate responsibility for patient care and ensuring that interventions were carried out and documented.

Whether delegating or simply coordinating care among a variety of health care team members, the RN must maintain a level of professionalism and respect when interacting with everyone. To provide the best patient-centered care, all team members must take their responsibilities seriously. The nurse's attitude and actions when interacting with others impact their feelings, which can have a tremendous effect on how care is delivered.

Effects of Collaboration in Health Care on Patient Safety and Positive Patient Outcomes LO 4.3

Patient safety is enhanced when there is a collaborative effort among health care team members. Patient injury, prolonged hospitalization, and accidental death are prevented when medication administration procedures are followed in collaboration with several members of the interdisciplinary team. Injuries from falls are avoided when all staff members who come in contact with a patient follow fall precautions. The spread of infection is inhibited when nurses educate patients, families, and other staff members about proper isolation precautions.

Many health care providers, including the prescribing physician or nurse practitioner, pharmacist, respiratory therapist, dietitian, and nurse, collaborate for the safe administration of medications. In consultation with the prescribing provider, the pharmacist ensures that the correct medication is sent to the patient unit. The dietitian may evaluate the patient's diet to confirm that it enhances a medication's desired effects. Respiratory therapists often administer inhaled medications. Nurses have the specialized knowledge and are often the final professional involved before a medication is administered, making them the last line of defense against errors. Many facilities require nurses to prepare medication in a No Interruption Zone focusing only on preparing the correct medication. Nurses are also responsible for patient education concerning medications, side effects, and administration requirements. Multidisciplinary collaboration for medication administration helps safeguard against errors.

Positive patient outcomes are best promoted through the use of a multidisciplinary care team. The occupational

---

Box 4.4 Examples of Interventions That Can and Cannot Be Delegated to Unlicensed Assistive Personnel

Interventions That Can Be Delegated Following the Five Rights of Delegation	Interventions That Cannot Be Delegated
• Routine vital sign assessment of stable patients	• Assessment
• Hygienic care such as bathing, shampooing, oral care, and bedmaking	• Care Planning
• Back massage	• Development of a patient teaching plan
• Toileting	• Changing dressings on acute wounds
• Turning and positioning of patients	• Irrigating a wound
• Range-of-motion exercises	• Collecting a wound culture or a urine specimen from a catheter
• Assistance with ambulation	• Tracheostomy, nasotracheal or nasopharyngeal suctioning of a patient
• Application of antiembolism hose or sequential compression devices	• Care of a new tracheostomy
• Changing a simple nonsterile dressing on an established wound in some facilities	• Care of chest tubes
• Application of wraps, bandages, or binders	• Changing the pouch of a new ostomy, or care of an ostomy with complications
• Collecting sputum, stool, and voided urine specimens.	• Inserting a Foley catheter
• Blood glucose testing	• Bladder irrigation
• Oral and oropharyngeal suctioning	• Medication administration
• Care of an established tracheostomy	• Starting and maintaining a peripheral intravenous injection
• Changing the pouch or care of an ostomy without complications	• Patient education
	• Discharge instruction

---

therapist evaluates the safety of patient performance of ADL and recommends equipment and supplies that can enhance patient safety. The evaluation of ambulation is carried out by the physical therapist who makes recommendation for assistive devices such as canes or walkers to promote patient safety when ambulating. The social worker facilitates contact with insurance companies or other agencies to assist with the financing of recommended therapeutic assistive and specialty devices. Under the delegation of the RN, UAP provide hands-on care for patients who require assistance with ADL, transfers, and ambulation. To prevent pressure ulcers in a bed-ridden patient, the nurse works with the dietitian to ensure proper nutrition and with UAP to establish a turning schedule.

Collaboration of the interdisciplinary health care team is essential to meeting the common goal of quality patient care. Planning comprehensive, collaborative care that addresses the multiple needs of patients often facilitates shorter recovery or rehabilitation periods, leading to reduced length of hospitalization and greater patient satisfaction. Carrying out interventions and meeting patient needs is often dependent on involvement from several members of the team working cooperatively. Knowing when and how to delegate and work collaboratively are vital skills for the nurse to possess.

REFERENCES

Cronenwett L, Sherwood G, Barnsteiner J, et al. Quality and safety education for nurses. *Nurs Outlook*. 2007;55(3):122–131.

Sullivan M, Kiovsky R, Mason D, et al. Interprofessional collaboration and education. *Am J Nurs*. 2015;115(3):47–54.

CHAPTER 5

Critical Thinking

Learning Outcomes

Comprehension of this chapter's content will provide students with the ability to:

LO 5.1   Identify the components necessary for critical thinking.

LO 5.2   Discuss the role of critical thinking in nursing practice.

LO 5.3   Explain methods for improving critical thinking skills.

Critical thinking is integral to all aspects of professional nursing practice. Critical thinking involves analysis of information, thoughtful interpretation and synthesis of ideas, and the rethinking of assumptions. Nursing requires this type of higher-order thinking so that nurses can accurately assess and analyze clinical issues and make sound clinical judgments and decisions. According to Benner, Sutphen, Leonard, and Day (2010), nursing education at all levels requires active participation of students in the classroom and lab, and the integration of theory and practice to facilitate the development of strong critical thinking and clinical reasoning skills. For the nurse, critical thinking provides a framework for reflection on judgments and actions that can improve patient outcomes and increase the accuracy of clinical decisions. Professional nursing practice requires a commitment to compassion, competency, and collaboration, and involves autonomy and accountability that make sound critical thinking essential for safe patient care.

Components of Critical Thinking   LO 5.1

Critical thinking has become a buzzword for all types of thinking, but it must be differentiated from casual or haphazard thinking, such as trial and error. Nurses make life-and-death decisions on the basis of critical thinking influenced by scientific research and best practices. Critical thinking is not random or casual thinking. It requires an overall desire to learn and involves specific components

including a strong knowledge base, and skill in reasoning, inference, and validation (Fig. 5.1).

Knowledge Review

Because critical thinking is disciplined, it is contextual and requires knowledge of the subject on which thought is taking place. It is not possible for a person to critically think about something about which the person has no knowledge. For example, critical thinking is used by nurses to guide decisions related to responsibilities such as delegation of assignments and tasks to unlicensed assistive personnel (UAP). Before delegation of a task, the nurse must be knowledgeable about the role, scope of practice, and competency of the recipient of the delegated task.

Information Gathering

Data collection during the assessment process is an important component of information gathering. Often the focus of data collection is based on knowledge gaps, missing patient information that would clarify the patient's situation. The application of critical-thinking skills to information gathering assists the nurse in collecting relevant, precise, and accurate patient data. Because clinical decisions are often based on the data that is collected, it is important that the nurse uses critical-thinking skills during assessment.

Nurses must be equipped with a large knowledge base in addition to data collection and information-gathering skills to help find answers when faced with new problems, questions, and situations. To respond to challenges that emerge, nurses must gather information on research findings related to the situation with which they are faced. Research findings, combined with patient values and needs, clinical competence, and cost-effectiveness comprise evidence-based practice. Reading professional journals, participating in professional organizations, attending continuing education events, and conducting literature reviews and research appropriate to their practice settings are some of the information gathering methods nurses can use to develop stronger critical thinking skills (Fig. 5.2).

Reasoning

Reasoning is a formal method of thinking that seeks to find answers to a problem or come to a decision on a challenging topic. Nurses use clinical reasoning to monitor patients through ongoing assessment and evaluation and to guide decision making. Nurses use both inductive reasoning and deductive reasoning in their practice. Inductive reasoning uses specific facts or details to draw conclusions and generalizations; it proceeds from specific to general. Deductive

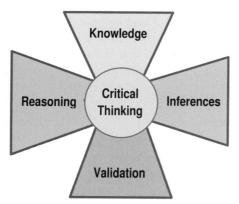

FIG. 5.1 Components of critical thinking.

reasoning involves generating facts or details from a major theory, generalization, or premise (i.e., from general to specific). Both types of reasoning can be beneficial in thinking critically about challenging clinical situations.

Inferences

Inferences are conclusions based on some type of information or experience. The accuracy of an inference is directly related to the correctness of what the inference is based on. Inferences are frequently based on assumptions, which are beliefs that are taken for granted and presumed to be true. Assumptions may be used erroneously to guide decision making when they are based on something that was previously learned and not questioned. It is important that nurses examine their assumptions and inferences about patients and their health care. Inferences may be logical or illogical, accurate or inaccurate, justified or unjustified. Nurses must question their assumptions to avoid making inferences that negatively impact patient care.

Intuition

Intuition is the feeling that something is known without specific evidence. Intuition is gaining favor as a valid characteristic of expert clinical judgment acquired through knowledge, practice, and experience. Alfaro-LeFevre (2017) explains that expert nurses use intuition to facilitate problem solving because their hunches (most likely intuition) are based on experiential knowledge. Less experienced nurses rely more on logic and a step-by-step approach when encountering the same issue (Fig. 5.3). In either situation, intuition based on critical thinking requires analysis and evidence to support actions.

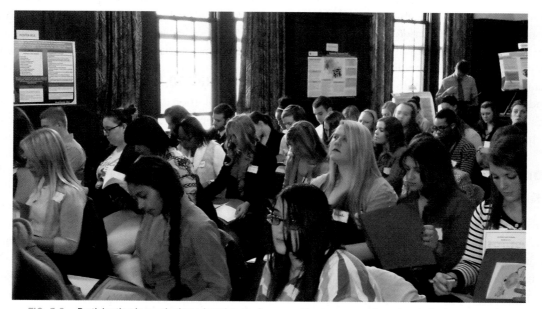

FIG. 5.2 Participating in continuing education conferences allows nurses and nursing students to expand their knowledge base and support higher levels of critical thinking.

Interpretation

Examining how information is organized and given meaning guides the interpretation of the information. Interpretations must be differentiated from facts and evidence because they are based on personal conceptions, experiences, and perspective. Interpretation of data is an important aspect of professional nursing practice. Some data are objective (e.g., laboratory values, diagnostic examination results, clinical manifestations), and other data are subjective (e.g., facial expressions, mood, body language). However, in both situations, nurses are expected to interpret data and use it to guide their decisions and actions.

Validation

Along with the specific components of critical thinking—knowledge, reasoning, and inferences—validation of information is required before taking action. Alfaro-LeFevre (2017) defines validation as checking accuracy and reliability. One aspect of validation is to find support for the findings or data. As was mentioned in Chapter 2, subjective data (Patient states, "I feel tired all of the time.") can sometimes be validated with objective data (low hemoglobin indicating anemia).

The Role of Critical Thinking in Nursing Practice   LO 5.2

The rapid rate of change and increasing complexity of health care and information technology make critical thinking essential in nursing. No longer is rote memorization and recall of content sufficient for the complex decisions and judgment required in professional nursing practice. Because knowledge and technology continue to expand for nursing professionals, the content learned in nursing school is not sufficient to maintain competence in nursing practice.

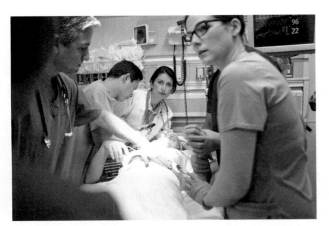

FIG. 5.3   The intuition and knowledge of experienced nurses can help direct the practice of newer colleagues in emergency situations.

Professional nursing requires a commitment to lifelong learning. Nurses must possess critical-thinking skills to maintain pace with ever-changing treatment modalities and technological advances. It is an expectation of professional practice that nurses maintain competency and update their knowledge base throughout their careers. Maintaining competency through professional development and reviewing research is facilitated by having critical-thinking abilities. Because nursing requires the application of knowledge to make clinical decisions and guide care, it involves active participation by the nurse. The application of knowledge requires development of a questioning attitude. This process is sometimes referred to as *thinking like a nurse*. Fig. 5.4 provides critical thinking examples utilized by nurses and nursing students outside and within the clinical setting (Alfaro-LaFevre, 2017).

Methods for Improving Critical Thinking Skills   LO 5.3

Improved critical thinking skills come with practice and intentional effort. Just as developing psychomotor skills (i.e., giving injections, placing a urinary catheter) require time to perfect, advanced critical thinking skills involve a commitment of time and effort to acquire. Multiple strategies are available to nurses to improve their critical thinking skills.

Reflection

Reflecting on thoughts, ideas, actions, and experiences provides individuals, including nurses, with the opportunity to gain insight into the validity and value of those thoughts or actions. Reflection may allow an individual to develop creative ideas for problem solving or to change unhealthy or destructive behaviors. Reflection is especially helpful to nurses because it allows for investigation of best practices and openness to new ways of thinking. It requires a commitment of time and is an essential aspect of critical thinking and professional growth. Although reflection is typically an activity undertaken in solitude, many strategies that build critical thinking skills are more interactive.

Discussion with Colleagues

Discussion of a problem, issue, or situation with colleagues may improve critical thinking. Through dialogue with others who have expertise or experience with the issue being faced, knowledge gaps can be filled, erroneous assumptions exposed, and unconscious biases addressed. Nurses can verify their assessments and diagnoses through discussion with colleagues to enhance clarity and accuracy (Fig. 5.5).

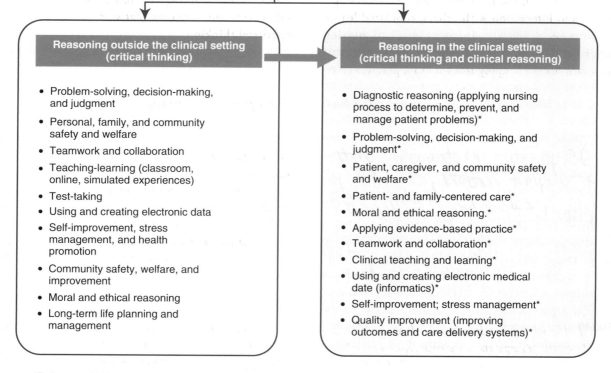

CRITICAL THINKING	
Reasoning outside the clinical setting (critical thinking)	**Reasoning in the clinical setting (critical thinking and clinical reasoning)**
• Problem-solving, decision-making, and judgment • Personal, family, and community safety and welfare • Teamwork and collaboration • Teaching-learning (classroom, online, simulated experiences) • Test-taking • Using and creating electronic data • Self-improvement, stress management, and health promotion • Community safety, welfare, and improvement • Moral and ethical reasoning • Long-term life planning and management	• Diagnostic reasoning (applying nursing process to determine, prevent, and manage patient problems)* • Problem-solving, decision-making, and judgment* • Patient, caregiver, and community safety and welfare* • Patient- and family-centered care* • Moral and ethical reasoning.* • Applying evidence-based practice* • Teamwork and collaboration* • Clinical teaching and learning* • Using and creating electronic medical date (informatics)* • Self-improvement; stress management* • Quality improvement (improving outcomes and care delivery systems)*

*Relates to ANA practice standards, The Joint Commission Standards, Quality and Safety Education for Nurses competencies, and National Academy of Medicine competencies

FIG. 5.4 Critical thinking is used by nurses repeatedly in their daily lives and while practicing nursing.

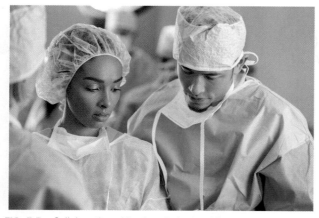

FIG. 5.5 Collaborating with others helps provide a new perspective in challenging patient care situations.

Audible Verbalization of Thoughts

Sometimes processing information out loud can help to clarify a situation and provide critical insights. By verbally examining patient or circumstantial data, assumptions, or plans for their accuracy and relevance, nurses may uncover solutions to complex situations. Processing information audibly incorporates elements of reflection while moving beyond examining only personal thoughts.

Literature Review

Because critical thinking cannot occur about subjects that are unknown, a review of literature can help to alleviate knowledge deficits. The process of literature review is organized and logical by nature. The more accurate, clear, and precise nurses can be in approaching the literature, the greater the likelihood that the information discovered will address the original issue, question, or problem.

Intentional Application of Knowledge

Nursing practice is based on the application of knowledge to address patient problems. Case studies that present patient scenarios, such as the ones presented in this book, provide nurses and students with basic and more complex situations that require the application of critical thinking skills. Case studies use problem-based learning that focuses on solving real-world problems. They are a valuable method of improving critical thinking. Once case studies are explored, the insights and knowledge gained can be applied in the clinical setting to provide safer, evidence-based, patient-centered care.

Simulation

Because critical thinking skills involve knowledge, reflection, and interaction with others, simulated learning environments are a tremendous asset to nursing education and practice. Simulated experiences permit nurses and students to apply information, practice complicated interventions, or experiment with new technologies in a safe and realistic environment that allows time for questions, clarification, and feedback (Fig. 5.6). Simulation exercises provide opportunities for nurses to explore their thinking and reflect on the assumptions, inferences, and decisions that were made—all elements of critical thinking.

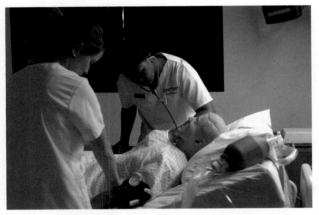

FIG. 5.6 Simulation lab experiences challenge students to synthesize and apply their knowledge to patient care in a safe environment.

Concept Maps

Concept maps are widely used in education and business to visually identify relationships and solve problems. Although many types of concepts maps exist, they are most often diagrams that show relationships between data using various shapes, lines, and arrows (Fig. 5.7). Nurses and nursing students often use concept maps to help understand the relationship between disease pathophysiology and treatment. Sometimes visualizing concepts in relationship to others on paper or electronically facilitates greater comprehension and improved critical thinking and clinical decision-making.

Conceptual Care Maps

Throughout this book, conceptual care maps (CCMs) are used to assist the reader to organize assessment data and apply critical-thinking skills to the development

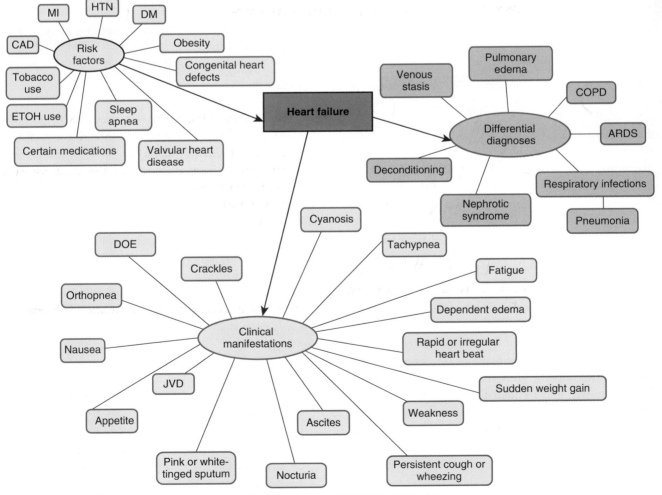

FIG. 5.7 Concept maps are visual tools that display relationships among data.

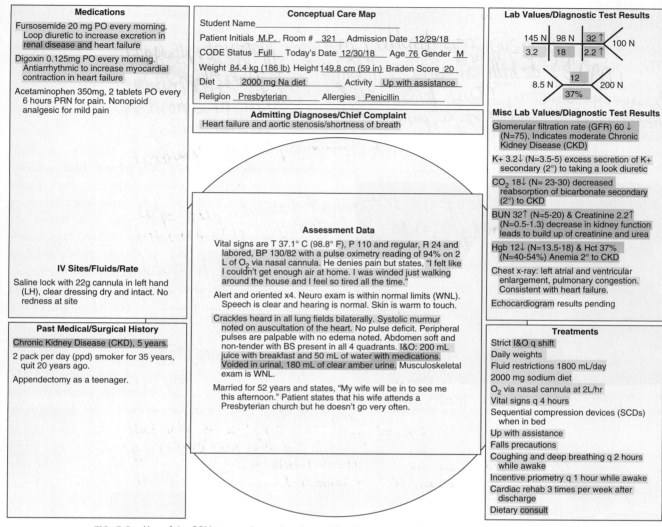

Medications

Fursosemide 20 mg PO every morning. Loop diuretic to increase excretion in renal disease and heart failure

Digoxin 0.125mg PO every morning. Antiarrhythmic to increase myocardial contraction in heart failure

Acetaminophen 350mg, 2 tablets PO every 6 hours PRN for pain. Nonopioid analgesic for mild pain

IV Sites/Fluids/Rate

Saline lock with 22g cannula in left hand (LH), clear dressing dry and intact. No redness at site

Past Medical/Surgical History

Chronic Kidney Disease (CKD), 5 years.

2 pack per day (ppd) smoker for 35 years, quit 20 years ago.

Appendectomy as a teenager.

Conceptual Care Map

Student Name_____

Patient Initials _M.P._ Room # _321_ Admission Date _12/29/18_

CODE Status _Full_ Today's Date _12/30/18_ Age _76_ Gender _M_

Weight _84.4 kg (186 lb)_ Height _149.8 cm (59 in)_ Braden Score _20_

Diet _____2000 mg Na diet_____ Activity _Up with assistance_

Religion _Presbyterian_ Allergies _Penicillin_

Admitting Diagnoses/Chief Complaint

Heart failure and aortic stenosis/shortness of breath

Assessment Data

Vital signs are T 37.1° C (98.8° F), P 110 and regular, R 24 and labored, BP 130/82 with a pulse oximetry reading of 94% on 2 L of O_2 via nasal cannula. He denies pain but states, "I felt like I couldn't get enough air at home. I was winded just walking around the house and I feel so tired all the time."

Alert and oriented x4. Neuro exam is within normal limits (WNL). Speech is clear and hearing is normal. Skin is warm to touch.

Crackles heard in all lung fields bilaterally. Systolic murmur noted on auscultation of the heart. No pulse deficit. Peripheral pulses are palpable with no edema noted. Abdomen soft and non-tender with BS present in all 4 quadrants. I&O: 200 mL juice with breakfast and 50 mL of water with medications. Voided in urinal, 180 mL of clear amber urine. Musculoskeletal exam is WNL.

Married for 52 years and states, "My wife will be in to see me this afternoon." Patient states that his wife attends a Presbyterian church but he doesn't go very often.

Lab Values/Diagnostic Test Results

145 N | 98 N | 32 ↑ | 100 N
3.2 | 18 | 2.2 ↑

8.5 N | 12 | 200 N
37%

Misc Lab Values/Diagnostic Test Results

Glomerular filtration rate (GFR) 60 ↓ (N=75), Indicates moderate Chronic Kidney Disease (CKD)

K+ 3.2↓ (N=3.5-5) excess secretion of K+ secondary (2°) to taking a look diuretic

CO_2 18↓ (N= 23-30) decreased reabsorption of bicarbonate secondary (2°) to CKD

BUN 32↑ (N=5-20) & Creatinine 2.2↑ (N=0.5-1.3) decrease in kidney function leads to build up of creatinine and urea

Hgb 12↓ (N=13.5-18) & Hct 37% (N=40-54%) Anemia 2° to CKD

Chest x-ray: left atrial and ventricular enlargement, pulmonary congestion. Consistent with heart failure.

Echocardiogram results pending

Treatments

Strict I&O q shift

Daily weights

Fluid restrictions 1800 mL/day

2000 mg sodium diet

O_2 via nasal cannula at 2L/hr

Vital signs q 4 hours

Sequential compression devices (SCDs) when in bed

Up with assistance

Falls precautions

Coughing and deep breathing q 2 hours while awake

Incentive priometry q 1 hour while awake

Cardiac rehab 3 times per week after discharge

Dietary consult

FIG. 5.8 Use of the CCM to organize and analyze patient data supports the enhancement of critical thinking skills.

of care plans and patient care. CCMs require the nurse to organize, cluster, analyze, and synthesize data while identifying relationships among findings. This learning and organizational tool assists in the development of patient-centered goals, the recognition of evidence-based research interventions, and the evaluation of patient outcomes. The CCM is a visual representation of the nurse's critical-thinking process and patient care plan (Fig. 5.8).

Critical thinking is required to complete each of the case studies presented as *patient assignments* in this book. As discussed, critical thinking is essential for safe, effective, professional nursing practice. It facilitates the collection of accurate patient data and the planning of patient-centered, evidence-based nursing care. Critical thinking is a skill that can be improved and facilitated through intentional and consistent application. Integrated into the nursing process, critical thinking is the method through which nurses *think*

like a nurse. It supports the transformation of a student into the professional nursing role.

Take time to develop or refine the critical thinking skills needed for professional nursing practice by working through each of the *patient assignments* presented. Aspects of risk, etiology and disease processes, patient-centered care, prevention, patient education, communication, referral, support, delegation, collaboration, research, and safety as well as many other factors are integrated into the *patient assignments* within the case study and CCM frameworks. Be prepared to learn and grow professionally while developing greater skills in communication, collaboration, and care.

REFERENCES

Alfaro-LeFevre R. *Critical thinking, clinical reasoning, and clinical judgment: A practical approach*, 6th ed. St. Louis: Elsevier; 2017.

Benner P, Sutphen M, Leonard V, et al. *Educating nurses: A call for radical transformation*. San Francisco: Jossey-Bass; 2010.

CASE STUDY 1

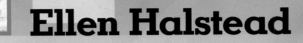

Ellen Halstead

Name/s _Quynh Le_   **Date** _04/29/2016_

Patient Assignment

E.H. is an 84-year-old female newly admitted to the hospital with a diagnosis of r/o pneumonia. She is recently widowed and lives alone. This is the first time E.H. has been in the hospital since she delivered her youngest child. She plays tennis three times a week and is in excellent physical condition. All three of her children live out of town but are in contact with her via phone or email several times each week.

Initial Assessment

37°C Normal.   _120/80 60-100_   _95._

1110 VS: T (39.5° C) (103.2° F), BP 102/58, P 88 and regular, R 36 and labored. O$_2$ saturation 88% on RA. E.H. reports her pain level as 2/10 when she "gets a coughing jag"; otherwise, her pain is 0/10. She is A&O×4, PERRLA. Lung sounds reveal bilateral crackles with a nonproductive cough. Apical pulse is 88 and regular. Abdomen is soft with bowel sounds in all four quadrants. No dependent edema. Pedal pulses +2 bilaterally.

Admission Orders

Admit to medical unit, vital signs q4 hr with O$_2$ sat; administer and titrate oxygen 2 to 4 L via NC to maintain O$_2$ sat >90%, sputum specimen, CBC, BMP, chest x-ray, saline lock, I&O, adult regular diet, up *ad lib*

1. Identify at least four potential causes of pneumonia.

Virus, bacteria, mycoplasma organisms, fungi
poarasites, & chemicals

amonia | expect WBC ↑

2. List a minimum of seven risk factors that increase a person's susceptibility to pneumonia. Highlight or circle the one(s) that E.H. possesses.

Upper respiratory infection, altered conciousness, prolonged bedrest, or immobility, chronic illness (COPD), chronic bronchitis, environmental factor, immunodepressive disease, feeding tube, malnutrition, living or traveling in high density situation, intubation.

3. Identify assessment factors that indicated the possible need for E.H. to be hospitalized.

age 84, elevated temperature, respiratory rate of 36 & labored, O_2 saturation of 88% on room temperature, blood pressure of 102/58, bilateral crackles, non productive cough

4. Write a minimum of eight assessment questions that would be most beneficial to ask E.H. to help determine the cause of her admission diagnosis of r/o pneumonia.

Are you aware of having been exposed to any one with pneumonia. were you painted or cleaning w/ any caustic solution that you are aware Did you get flu shot this year Have you ever had pneumonia before. Have you had pneumonia vaccine. Did you have acold before developing your labored breathing.

5. What laboratory and diagnostic findings will verify that E.H. has pneumonia? Explain how those findings will lead to the diagnosis of pneumonia.

- elevated WBC (>15,000 uL) revealing an infection & ↑ chest x ray indicating the presence of infiltrate will verify the diagnosis of pneumonia.
- A sputum culture can help to identify the causative organism allowing for more specific antibiotic therapy if the pneumonia is bacterial.

6. What three nursing interventions are your highest priorities? Provide a rationale for your actions.

elevate E.H.'s head of bed to assist w/ her eased of breathing, initiate oxygen therapy @ 2 L per nasal cannula (NC) & monitor her O_2 saturation to maintain it @ or above 90%.

7. On what will your focused assessments on E.H. concentrate?

- Respiratory assessment . respiratory rate & effort , shortness of breath, dyspnea or exertion , oxygen saturation , lung auscultation, cough & septum production
- vital signs including pain assessment.
- level of conciousness & alertness .
- intake & out put .

8. What classifications of medication would you anticipate being ordered for E.H. after it is determined that she has bacterial pneumonia? Provide a brief rationale for administering each one.

Antibiotics - to treat the infection (pneumonia) .

Antipyretics - to treat fever .

Analgesic - to treat pain

9. Of the three nursing diagnoses labels listed, which is the highest priority for E.H. at this time? Highlight or circle your answer and provide a rationale.

q?

Acute pain
Impaired gas exchange (highest priority for EH @ this time bc her oxygen satr is blow 90% on room air . It requires immediate intervention to avoid having her respiratory effort worsen .
Risk for falls

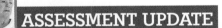

ASSESSMENT UPDATE

By the next morning at 0750, E.H.'s temperature has fallen to 38.5° C (101.3° F) and her O_2 saturation is staying at only 92% on 2 L of oxygen. Unfortunately, she appears increasingly SOB and her lung sounds include minor expiratory wheezing and course crackles on auscultation. E.H. is coughing more frequently and having difficulty expelling thick, yellowish sputum.

10. What additional PCP orders would you anticipate for E.H. today?

Aerosol breathing treatment by respiratory therapist.

11. You notice that E.H.'s output has exceeded her intake for the past 24 hours. What do you suggest to her PCP during rounds and what do you suggest to E.H.?

↑ IV fluid rate would be one way to increase E.H.'s intake that would be require an order from the primary care provider. Increased oral intake of fluid can be beneficial to help thin secretion. This would be especially bc she is having difficulty expelling thick sputum.

12. Of the three nursing diagnosis labels listed, which is the highest priority for E.H. now? Highlight or circle your answer and provide a rationale.

Impaired gas exchange
Fluid volume deficit
Ineffective airway clearance is the highest nursing priority or E.H bc of inability to expell thick sputum, which appears to be contributing to narrowed air way & more effort for breathing

13. Complete a nursing care plan on the CCM for Case Study 1 in this book or in the CCM Creator on Evolve for the two identified nursing diagnoses based on E.H.'s assessment findings during her hospitalization. Include a minimum of two to three nursing interventions to address each short-term goal (STG) that you identify. Refer to Chapter 1 of this book as needed for guidance in completing your work.

See (Concept map care).

ASSESSMENT UPDATE

Three days after her admission, vital signs for E.H. are within normal limits (WNL) and she is responding to antibiotic therapy. Her O_2 sat is 96% on RA, her sputum production is significantly less and she is able to cough up her secretions without difficulty. E.H. is able to walk on the unit without any SOB.

14. What are some discharge instructions that you should provide for E.H.?

Discharge instructions may included w/o being limited to

- Complete the order antibiotic therapy even if you begin to feel much better before all of the med is gone.
- Rest between activities, & then resume your normal activities when you fell strong enough w/o any shortness of breath
- limit yr exposure to others may be ill
- drink plenty of fluids & eat a heathy, balanced diet.
- Get a flu shot & or pneumonial vaccine after you have fully recovered per recommendation of ur PCP.
- follow up w/ ur PCP @ the recommendation time.

Medications

IV Sites/Fluids/Rate

Past Medical/Surgical History

Conceptual Care Map

Student Name _____

Patient Initials __E.H.__ Room # _____ Admission Date _____

CODE Status _____ Today's Date _____

Age __84__ Gender __F__ Weight _____ Height ____ Braden Score _____

Diet __Adult regular_____ Activity __Up ad lib_____

Religion _____ Allergies _____

Admitting Diagnoses/Chief Complaint
R/O pneumonia

Assessment Data

Initial Assessment:

1110 VS: 39° C (103.2° F), BP 102/58, P 88 and regular, R 36 and labored. O_2 saturation 88% on RA. Pt. reports pain level of 0/10 normally and 2/10 when she "gets a coughing jag."

A&Ox4, PERRLA

Crackles bilaterally with nonproductive cough. Apical 88 and regular. Abdomen soft with BS in all four quadrants. No dependent edema. Pedal pulses 2+ bilaterally.

Assessment Update:

0750 VS: 38.5° C (101.3° F), O_2 sat 93% on 2 L per NC. Increased SOB, minor expiratory wheezing and coarse crackles bilaterally. Increased cough. Difficulty expelling thick, yellowish sputum

Lab Values/Diagnostic Test Results

BMP

CBC

Misc Lab Values/Diagnostic Test Results

Treatments

VS q4 hr with O_2 sat

Titrate oxygen 2-4 L via NC to maintain O_2 sat >90%

Sputum culture

CBC

BMP

Chest x-ray

Saline lock

I&O

Primary Nursing Diagnosis	Nursing Diagnosis 2	Nursing Diagnosis 3
Supporting Data	Supporting Data	Supporting Data
STG/NOC	STG/NOC	STG/NOC
Interventions/NIC with Rationale	Interventions/NIC with Rationale	Interventions/NIC with Rationale
Rationale Citation/EBP	Rationale Citation/EBP	Rationale Citation/EBP
Evaluation	Evaluation	Evaluation

ⒺAn interactive version of the Conceptual Care Map is on Evolve.

CASE STUDY

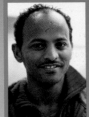

2

Jamaal Samatar

Name/s _____ Date _____

Patient Assignment

J.S. is a 28-year-old Somalian who lived in a refugee camp for 2 years before moving to live with family abroad 3 months ago. He has had a persistent cough for the past month and is waking up at night sweating. When he arrives at the community health clinic and shares his symptoms with the triage nurse, the nurse immediately initiates appropriate isolation precautions and makes arrangements for J.S. to be admitted to the acute care medical center on your nursing unit for further assessment and treatment of suspected tuberculosis.

Initial Assessment

1024 VS: T 38.8° C (101.8° F), BP 132/78, P 68 and regular, R 24 and unlabored. O_2 saturation 92% on RA. J.S. reports a persistent pain level of 3/10 stating that the pain is in his chest and "tight," nonradiating in nature. J.S. is A&O×4, PERRLA, with no JVD on admission. His lungs have fine crackles bilaterally on auscultation, and he struggles to cough up thick "reddish" sputum. Bowel sounds are present in all four quadrants, MAE, with 2+ pedal pulses and no dependent edema.

1. List three risk factors for developing active tuberculosis (TB) after contracting the *M. tuberculosis* bacterium.

2. Identify symptoms of active infection with *M. tuberculosis* bacterium.

3. List the risk factors and symptoms that J.S. has that led the triage nurse to suspect tuberculosis.

4. TB is spread person-to-person when an individual with active TB speaks, coughs, or sneezes releasing miniscule droplets into the air. As the nurse caring for J.S. when he is admitted, what type of room placement should you initiate?

5. Describe the type of isolation that J.S. should be placed in, where signage should be placed, and the corresponding requirements for care givers and the patient.

6. As the admitting nurse, identify a minimum of five assessment topics or areas on which to ask questions about and focus on during your initial physical examination of J.S.

7. What initial diagnostic tests would typically be ordered for J.S.?

8. Based on initial assessment findings for J.S., what nursing diagnoses would you identify for him? Enter your top two nursing diagnoses into the CCM for Case Study 2 in this book or in the CCM Creator on Evolve to begin the development of his patient-centered plan of care. Be sure to include a *related to* (r/t) statement and list supporting data *as evidenced by* (aeb) from the assessment findings for each diagnosis.

ASSESSMENT UPDATE

Forty-eight hours postadmission, diagnostic tests confirm that J.S. has active pulmonary tuberculosis. Additional nursing assessment findings include weight loss of 10 lb in the past month, daily consumption of less than 50% of his meals, occasional O_2 saturation levels of 88% on RA, DOE noted when ambulating to the bathroom, continued intermittent productive cough.

9. Given J.S.'s admission and these additional assessment findings, what nursing interventions and prescribed treatments do you as the nurse anticipate integrating into J.S.'s plan of care? List a minimum of seven.

10. List a minimum of three other members of the interdisciplinary health care team that you as the primary nurse for J.S. may collaborate with during his hospitalization. Briefly explain each person's role in his care.

11. Add an additional nursing diagnosis or patient problem to your CCM with its etiology and supporting data. Write short-term goals for all three of the nursing diagnoses you have identified and list associated interventions with rationales for each. Fill in additional assessment and treatment data as needed.

12. The core drug regimen for treating TB is isoniazid (INH), rifampin (RIF), ethambutol (EMB), and pyrazinamide (PZA) for 6 to 9 months. It is vitally important for patients to take their medications exactly as they are prescribed for the entire period of time needed. Identify at least two reasons for patients to take their TB medications for the entire period of time as prescribed.

13. Identify life-threatening side effects for each of the TB drugs, including isoniazid (INH), rifampin (RIF), ethambutol (EMB), and pyrazinamide (PZA). For each drug, list the reactions that patients should be instructed to report to their PCP.

14. Provide evaluation statements for each of the short-term goals you identified in the nursing care plan for J.S.

ASSESSMENT UPDATE

J.S. began treatment for active TB while hospitalized on your nursing unit. No members of his family or close contacts tested positive for TB. He is now preparing for discharge into the community.

15. What specific precautions should you discuss with J.S. because he is being discharged on medications, while still potentially contagious for the next 2 to 3 weeks? List a minimum of five.

16. What interventions can be effective in supporting patient compliance with the long-term TB medication regimen after discharge from the hospital?

17. In addition to his PCP, with whom will J.S. communicate regularly regarding follow-up care after his discharge to home?

Medications

IV Sites/Fluids/Rate

Past Medical/Surgical History

Conceptual Care Map

Student Name_____

Patient Initials _J.S._ Room # _____ Admission Date _____

CODE Status __Full__ Today's Date _____

Age _28_ Gender _M_ Weight _____ Height _____ Braden Score____

Diet _____ Activity _____

Religion _____ Allergies _____

Admitting Diagnoses/Chief Complaint
R/O active pulmonary tuberculosis

Assessment Data

Initial Assessment:

1024 VS: T 38.8° C (101.8° F), BP 132/78, P 68 and regular, R 24 and unlabored. O_2 saturation 92% on RA. J.S. reports a persistent pain level of 3/10 stating that the pain is in his chest and "tight," nonradiating in nature. J.S. is A&Ox4, PERRLA, with no JVD on admission. Persistent cough for past month. His lungs have fine crackles bilaterally on auscultation, and he struggles to cough up thick "reddish" sputum. BS are present in all four quadrants, MAE, with 2+ pedal pulses and no dependent edema. Wakes up sweating during the night.

Refugee from Somalia, moved abroad to live with family 3 months ago.

Assessment Update:

Weight loss of 10 lb in the past month, daily consumption of less than 50% of meals, occasional O_2 saturation levels of 88% on RA, DOE noted when ambulating to the bathroom, continued intermittent productive cough.

Lab Values/Diagnostic Test Results

BMP

CBC

Misc Lab Values/Diagnostic Test Results

AFB sputum culture-positive for *M. tuberculosis* bacterium

Treatments

Primary Nursing Diagnosis	Nursing Diagnosis 2	Nursing Diagnosis 3
Supporting Data	**Supporting Data**	**Supporting Data**
STG/NOC	**STG/NOC**	**STG/NOC**
Interventions/NIC with Rationale	**Interventions/NIC with Rationale**	**Interventions/NIC with Rationale**
Rationale Citation/EBP	**Rationale Citation/EBP**	**Rationale Citation/EBP**
Evaluation	**Evaluation**	**Evaluation**

ⓔAn interactive version of the Conceptual Care Map is on Evolve.

CASE STUDY

3

Rachelle Wagner

Name/s _____ Date _____

Patient Assignment

R.W. is a 42-year-old African American executive assistant who comes to the outpatient clinic for a routine physical. During the intake interview, R.W. reveals that she is experiencing considerable job stress, has two young teenagers at home, and is providing care for her elderly grandparents with the help of her husband.

Initial Assessment

1730 VS: T 37.5° C (98.6° F), BP 158/88, P 84 and regular, R 20 and unlabored. R.W. denies any pain and has an O_2 saturation of 98% on RA. Height: 172.7 cm (68 in), weight: 88.5 kg (195 lb) with a BMI of 29.6. R.W. is A&O×4, PERRLA, apical pulse is 84, lung sounds are clear throughout all lobes, abdomen is soft and large, no distention, bowel sounds present in all four quadrants. Pedal pulses 2+ bilaterally. R.W. states that she tends to eat more when she is under stress and has gained several pounds in the last few months. She denies any urinary or bowel problems.

1. As the clinic nurse, you know that R.W. is hypertensive based on what initial physical assessment finding?

2. What is the scale for determining if an adult patient is hypertensive? What is R.W.'s hypertension stage?

3. What are the known risk factors for hypertension? Name at least seven.

4. List the risk factors R.W. has for hypertension.

5. What are some general health history questions and questions related to known risk factors that you should ask R.W.? Identify a minimum of five.

6. The nurse practitioner orders bloodwork on R.W. including a BMP, prealbumin, and total cholesterol, LDL, and HDL levels. What is the purpose of each of these laboratory tests? Provide a brief explanation of their relevance to R.W.'s current health status.

After R.W.'s labs are drawn, she is instructed to return to the clinic in 3 days to get her lab test results and a BP check. R.W. indicates that she needs to hurry home and can't stay at the clinic any longer. R.W. is told that at her next visit, options for the treatment of hypertension will be discussed.

R.W.'s lab results are within normal range with the exception of her total cholesterol which is 220 mg/dL; her HDL which is 45 mg/dL; and her LDL which is 146 mg/dL. When she arrives at the clinic for her follow-up care, she appears rushed and is checking her phone when you walk into the room to complete a focused assessment.

Follow-up clinic visit: VS: T 36.8° C (98.2° F), BP 156/90, P 80 and regular, R 22 and unlabored. She reports no pain and her O_2 sat is 99% on RA. Her lungs are clear, abdomen soft with BS x4. Pedal pulses are 2+ bilaterally. She has no edema.

When asked about how she has been feeling the past 3 days, R.W. tells you that she had a bad headache yesterday and she is really concerned as to whether she can keep taking care of her grandparents while she is working and trying to attend her teenagers' co-curricular activities after school.

7. The nurse practitioner orders hydrochlorothiazide 25 mg PO q AM and atorvastatin 30 mg PO qd for initial pharmaceutical treatment of R.W.'s hypertension and high cholesterol. Explain the classification and nursing implications associated with each of these medications. List concerns about which you should educate R.W. before she begins taking hydrochlorothiazide and atorvastatin.

8. List a minimum of three other classifications of medication that are commonly used concurrently (with diuretics such as hydrochlorothiazide), or alone to treat hypertension. Provide a brief explanation of how each one works using words that a patient would understand.

9. Enter R.W.'s three cholesterol related lab results and medication orders into the CCM for Case Study 3 in this book or in the CCM Creator on Evolve. If a lab result is abnormal, indicate if it is high or low with an arrow, provide the normal range, and give a brief rationale for its current level. Below each medication, provide the classification of the medication and why it has been prescribed for R.W.

10. Prioritize the three possible nursing diagnosis labels for R.W. listed below. Add *related to* (r/t) statements to each one (as appropriate) and *as evidenced by* (aeb) assessment findings in the supporting data section of the CCM.

    Overweight
    Deficient knowledge
    Stress overload

11. Write short-term goals (and/or NOC classifications) for each of the three nursing diagnoses.

12. List a minimum of three hypertension related topics and lifestyle changes that you will discuss with R.W. to address her lack of information about hypertension.

13. Revise each of the general topics you identified and reword each one as a specific intervention with a cited rationale to help R.W. achieve the short-term goal you wrote for the nursing diagnosis label of Deficient Knowledge.

14. Identify a minimum of three stress reduction strategy options that would be appropriate for you to discuss with R.W. What community resources (both individuals and facilities) could provide support for R.W. in an effort to reduce her stress level?

15. What special diet plan has been found beneficial to individuals diagnosed with hypertension? Name and briefly explain it as you would to R.W. while providing her patient education.

16. In your CCM, complete R.W.'s plan of care by listing nursing interventions under each short-term goal and writing potential evaluation statements for each nursing diagnosis.

Medications

IV Sites/Fluids/Rate

Past Medical/Surgical History

Conceptual Care Map

Student Name _____

Patient Initials __R.W.__ Room # _____ Admission Date _____

CODE Status __Full__ Today's Date _____

Age _42_ Gender _F_ Weight _88.5 kg (195 lb)_ Height _172.7 cm (68 in)_

Braden Score_____ Diet _____ Activity _____

Religion _____ Allergies _____NKDA_____

Admitting Diagnoses/Chief Complaint
Routine physical

Assessment Data
Initial assessment findings:
VS: T 37.5° C (98.6° F), BP 158/88, P 84 and regular, R 20 and unlabored. Pain 0/0
O_2 saturation of 98% on RA.
Height: 172.7 cm (68 in), weight: 88.5 kg (195 lb) with a BMI of 29.6.
A&Ox4, PERRLA, apical 84, lung sounds are clear throughout all lobes, abdomen is soft and large, no distention, BS present in all four quadrants. Pedal pulses 2+ bilaterally.
Verbalizes considerable job stress. Mother of two teenagers.
Provides care for her grandparents with help from husband. States that she tends to eat more when she is under stress. Has gained several pounds in the last few months. Denies any urinary or bowel problems.

Assessment Update:
Follow-up clinic visit
VS: T 36.8° C (98.2° F), BP 156/90, P 80 and regular, R 22 and unlabored. Reports no pain. O_2 sat is 99% on RA. Lungs are clear, abdomen soft with BS x4. Pedal pulses are 2+ bilaterally. She has no edema.
Appears rushed and is checking her phone at the beginning of follow-up visit.
Reports a bad headache previous day. Shares concern as to whether she can keep taking care of her grandparents while working and trying to attend children's activities.

Lab Values/Diagnostic Test Results

BMP

CBC

Misc Lab Values/Diagnostic Test Results

Treatments

Primary Nursing Diagnosis	Nursing Diagnosis 2	Nursing Diagnosis 3
Supporting Data	Supporting Data	Supporting Data
STG/NOC	STG/NOC	STG/NOC
Interventions/NIC with Rationale	Interventions/NIC with Rationale	Interventions/NIC with Rationale
Rationale Citation/EBP	Rationale Citation/EBP	Rationale Citation/EBP
Evaluation	Evaluation	Evaluation

ⓔAn interactive version of the Conceptual Care Map is on Evolve.

CASE STUDY

4

Victoria Litchfield

Name/s_____ Date_____

Patient Assignment

V.L. is a 36-year-old female admitted from the ED last night with a diagnosis of r/o DVT. She came to the ED complaining of pain and swelling in her right calf. V.L. has been married for 10 years and has no children. She works as an executive for a manufacturing company and often travels for work. V.L. recently returned from a business trip to Asia that included 14-hour flights each way. Past medical and surgical history includes an appendectomy at age 16. V.L. takes oral contraceptives for birth control. An ultrasound was performed of the right leg which showed a clot restricting blood flow in the right posterior tibial vein in the lower leg.

Admission Orders

Admit to medical unit, vital signs q 4 hr with O_2 sat; CBC, BMP, chest x-ray, aPTT q 4 hr, PT/INR daily, I&O, adult regular diet, ambulation with assistance. Start a continuous IV with heparin 25,000 units in 250 mL D_5W at a rate of 1000 units/hr, call PCP with q 4 hr aPTT results; warfarin PO, call PCP with daily PT/INR results for warfarin orders. Acetaminophen 500 mg, 2 tablets PO q 8 hr PRN for pain. She received her first dose of acetaminophen in the ED at 2200 and the IV heparin was started. Her first dose of warfarin 2 mg PO was given at 2200.

1. Which risk factors for DVT (also known as venous thromboembolism or VTE) does V.L. exhibit?

2. List at least 8 other factors that increase a patient's risk for developing a DVT.

3. The ultrasound results show a thrombus in V.L.'s right posterior tibial vein in her right calf. V.L. states that she does not understand how this happened because she is young and healthy, and asks what the PCP meant by "deep vein thrombosis." Explain to V.L. how a thrombus forms in language the patient can understand.

4. Which focused assessments are priorities when you begin caring for V.L.? Give rationales for each.

5. What are the drug classifications of heparin and warfarin? What is the rationale behind giving V.L. both of these medications?

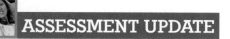

ASSESSMENT UPDATE

As the nurse assigned to care for V.L. the next morning, you receive report from the night nurse on your unit and proceed to complete morning assessments on your assigned patients. At 0730, V.L.'s morning assessment findings include: height 162.6 cm (64 in), weight 71.8 kg (158 lb). VS: T 36.5° C (97.7° F), BP 134/78, P 72 and regular, R 20 and unlabored. O₂ saturation 96% on RA. Apical pulse 74. V.L. states that the pain level in her right calf is 4/10 while lying still in bed. The pain is throbbing and she states that her pain level increases with any movement of the right leg to 7/10. She is A&Ox4. PERRLA. Lung sounds clear. Abdomen is soft and nontender with BS present in all 4 quadrants. MAE but guards right leg when moving. Nonpitting edema right lower leg. Pedal pulses 2+ on left and 1+ on right. Lower right leg is warm and tender. Right calf measures 41.5 cm compared with 38 cm on the left. Braden score 22. IV site with 22-g catheter in right forearm is patent and without redness or swelling. She has no known drug allergies and is a full code. V.L. states that she attends a Baptist church.

6. Begin to enter V.L.'s data into the CCM for Case Study 4 in this book or in the CCM Creator on Evolve. Include assessment data, lab results, treatments, and medications.

7. Using the initial and morning assessment information, list at least three nursing diagnoses or patient problems for V.L. Enter them into the CCM for Case Study 4 in this book or in the CCM Creator on Evolve to begin the development of her patient-centered plan of care.

8. What are your highest priority nursing interventions as you begin to care for V.L.?

9. As you monitor V.L.'s IV heparin drip, how many mL/hr will you set on the IV infusion pump?

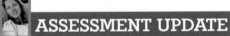

ASSESSMENT UPDATE

V.L. has been resting comfortably in bed and has ambulated to the bathroom twice with assistance. Her morning lab and test results include a normal CBC, BMP, and chest x-ray. Her aPTT is 60 seconds, and her PT results are 15 seconds with an INR of 1.4.

You call the PCP with these lab results and receive new orders: IV with heparin 25,000 units in 250 mL D$_5$W at a rate of 1100 units/hr, call PCP with q 4 hr aPTT results; warfarin 2 mg at 1800, call PCP with daily PT/INR results for further warfarin orders.

10. What is the new rate on the IV infusion pump?

11. What is the difference between the normal range of aPTT and the therapeutic values for patients taking heparin? What is the difference between the normal range of PT/INR and the therapeutic values for patients taking warfarin?

12. You are delegating part of V.L.'s care to an UAP. What interventions can be delegated to this member of the health care team? What special instructions should be given to the UAP before delegating care?

ASSESSMENT UPDATE

0730 on the second morning of V.L.'s hospitalization: pain level of 2/10 when resting and 4/10 with movement. She received acetaminophen before bedtime last night for pain of 4/10. VS: T 36.8° C (98.2° F), BP 128/76, P 68 and regular, R 20 and unlabored. O_2 saturation 98% on RA. Her right calf circumference is 40.5 cm, and her pedal pulses bilaterally are 2+ with slight nonpitting edema on the right. Her physical assessment is otherwise normal. V.L.'s lab results include: aPTT was 80 seconds, and her PT results were 18 seconds with an INR of 1.8.

You call the PCP with these lab results and receive new orders: Continue IV with heparin 25,000 units in 250 mL D_5W at a rate of 1100 units/hr, call PCP with q 4 hr aPTT results; warfarin 3 mg PO at 1800, call PCP with daily PT/INR results for further warfarin orders. Activity: Up ad lib.

13. Of the three nursing diagnoses or patient problems listed, which is the highest priority for V.L. at this time? Highlight or circle your answer and provide a rationale.

Acute pain

Ineffective peripheral tissue perfusion

Risk for bleeding

14. What is the rationale behind the activity order?

15. Finish completing the CCM for Case Study 4 in this book or in the CCM Creator on Evolve for the second day of V.L.'s hospitalization. Be sure to add the classification and rationale for each medication. Interpret all lab work listed on the CCM. When you group your supporting data, color code each piece to match the nursing diagnosis that corresponds with it. Include evaluation of the plan of care as of day 2 of hospitalization.

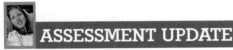

ASSESSMENT UPDATE

On the third morning V.L's vital signs are normal with a pain level of 2/10. She has 2+ pedal pulses bilaterally, and her right calf measurement is 39 cm. Lab results show an aPTT of 80 seconds, PT of 21 seconds and an INR of 2.5.

You call the PCP and receive new orders for V.L.: Discontinue IV heparin. Warfarin 3 mg PO today at 1800. Fit patient for thigh-high antiembolism hose. Discharge in the morning after the PT/INR results are called to PCP.

16. Explain why the heparin order was discontinued.

17. You discontinue the IV heparin, measure V.L. for thigh-high antiembolism hose, and begin discharge teaching. What instructions will be important to include in your teaching? Include information about anticoagulants, dietary considerations, and DVT prevention and reduction of risk factors.

18. Explain how to measure for thigh-high antiembolism hose.

Conceptual Care Map

Medications

IV Sites/Fluids/Rate

Past Medical/Surgical History

Student Name_____

Patient Initials __V.L.__ Room # _____ Admission Date _____

CODE Status _____ Today's Date _____ Age __36__ Gender __F__

Weight _____ Height _____

Braden Score____ Diet _____ Activity _____

Religion ____Baptist____ Allergies ____NKDA____

Admitting Diagnoses/Chief Complaint
R/O Deep Vein Thrombosis/Pain and swelling in right calf.

Assessment Data

Lab Values/Diagnostic Test Results

BMP

CBC

Misc Lab Values/Diagnostic Test Results

Treatments

Primary Nursing Diagnosis	Nursing Diagnosis 2	Nursing Diagnosis 3
Supporting Data	Supporting Data	Supporting Data
STG/NOC	STG/NOC	STG/NOC
Interventions/NIC with Rationale	Interventions/NIC with Rationale	Interventions/NIC with Rationale
Rationale Citation/EBP	Rationale Citation/EBP	Rationale Citation/EBP
Evaluation	Evaluation	Evaluation

ⓔAn interactive version of the Conceptual Care Map is on Evolve.

CASE STUDY

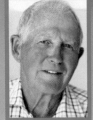

5

George Carlton

Name/s _____ Date _____

Patient Assignment

G.C. is a 76-year-old retired architect who was just admitted to a dementia unit in an extended care facility. He has a 4-year history of declining cognitive, psychosocial, and physical abilities. Past medical history includes hypertension for which he has taken metoprolol 50 mg PO bid for 8 years. He has taken memantine 5 mg PO bid for 3.5 years. G.C. is on an adult regular diet and is allowed up with supervision.

G.C.'s wife of 52 years has been his primary caregiver. She first noticed that something was different around 4 years ago when he started having trouble finding the word he wanted to say, and did not want to socialize with old friends or family. Around 3.5 years ago, he was diagnosed with Alzheimer disease. The disease has continued to progress to the point where his wife can no longer care for him by herself. He is often agitated and aggressive, and has wandered away from home several times.

1. What are the stages of Alzheimer disease (AD)? What are the clinical manifestations of each stage?

2. From your observations and his wife's descriptions of his behavior, in what stage of the disease is G.C.?

3. How is AD diagnosed?

4. What types of medications are available for Alzheimer patients?

5. Are there any focused assessment questions that you might ask his wife to better plan G.C.'s care?

ADMISSION ASSESSMENT

1100 VS: T 37° C (98.2° F), BP 132/84, P 64 and regular, R 24 and unlabored. O_2 saturation 98% on RA. G.C. does not respond to questions about pain. No wincing or crying out. He is A&O to person only. PERRLA. Lungs clear. Apical pulse is 64 and regular. Abdomen is soft with BS in all four quadrants. No dependent edema. Pedal pulses 2+ bilaterally. Skin is intact. Braden score is 19. He is 188 cm (74 in) tall and weighs 72.3 kg (170 lb). Ambulates slowly, often walking in the same pattern repeatedly. G.C. responds to his name, answers questions with unrelated comments, and repeats the same questions or statements over and over. He requires assistance of 1 for dressing, bathing, toileting, and oral care. His code status is DNR and he has NKDA.

G.C.'s wife tells you that he usually washes in the shower, but she has had to get into the shower with him lately because he doesn't know what to do when he is in the shower alone. He needs prompts to get dressed, and she helps him choose his clothes. She takes him to the bathroom every 2 to 3 hours when he is awake. He has not been eating well, so she has been trying to keep meals simple. She uses distraction and redirection when he becomes agitated. Music and television usually calm him. He likes to listen to oldies from the 1950s and 1960s and watches game shows on TV. He likes to draw with pencils or markers. He has been incontinent of urine a couple of times when they were away from home too long.

6. What is the first concern as you begin caring for G.C.?

7. Which interventions can you delegate to the UAP and LPN/LVN?

G.C.'s wife comes to visit 2 days after admission and shares that it has been a very difficult week. She is concerned about moving him to the facility. She says that she is exhausted but has not been able to sleep much in the couple of nights he has been here. Her three children are supportive, but they do not live close and are busy with jobs and raising their families. Most of their friends have disappeared from their lives in the past few years. She states that they even stopped going to their Congregational Church because it was too difficult with G.C. She feels badly if she does not visit him every day.

8. What support and suggestions can you offer or suggest to G.C.'s wife?

9. Which members of the interprofessional team might you collaborate with to provide information and support for G.C.'s wife?

10. Identify nursing diagnoses labels or patient problems for G.C. and his wife.

11. G.C. exhibits some behaviors such as aggression toward the staff, resisting care, repeatedly asking for his wife, and restlessness. As you plan his care, which interventions will help the staff deal with his behavior?

12. You have delegated G.C.'s shower to the UAP assigned to care for him. The UAP is experienced in working with Alzheimer patients but G.C. becomes combative when he is taken into the shower room. What can the UAP do to make the shower less frightening to G.C.?

13. Begin completing the CCM for Case Study 5 in this book or in the CCM Creator on Evolve for G.C. during the first few days he is in the extended care facility. Add pertinent data, cluster and highlight it, and prioritize three of the nursing diagnoses or patient problems that you identified in question 10. Be sure to add the classification and the reason why G.C. is taking each medication. Establish goals and interventions for each nursing diagnosis. Evaluate the plan of care at the end of this case study after G.C. has been in the facility for 3 weeks.

ASSESSMENT UPDATE

G.C. has now been in the facility for 3 weeks. His VS have been stable and his physical exam is unchanged. He does not eat all of his meals, and his weight is now 75.5 kg (166 lb). He is less agitated. He spends his days rocking in a chair in his room, wandering up and down the hallway, and doing drawings in the activity room. His wife visits about every other day and stays most of the day. You care for him several days per week.

14. What could account for his weight loss?

15. What are your priority assessments on an ongoing basis as you care for G.C.?

16. How have G.C.'s priority nursing diagnoses or patient problems changed after he has been in the facility for 3 weeks? List at least three nursing diagnoses or patient problems that are now the focus of your care plan for G.C. and his wife.

17. What are some priority interventions for G.C. now?

Medications

Metoprolol 50 mg PO bid
Memantine 5 mg PO bid

IV Sites/Fluids/Rate

Past Medical/Surgical History

Hypertension for 8 years
4-year history of declining cognitive, psychosocial, and physical abilities
Alzheimer disease 3.5 years

Conceptual Care Map

Student Name_____

Patient Initials _G.C._ Room # _____ Admission Date _____

CODE Status _DNR_ Today's Date _____ Age _76_ Gender _M_

Weight _72.3 kg (179 lb)_____ Height _188 cm (74 in)_____

Braden Score _19_ Diet _Adult regular_ Activity __Up with supervision__

Religion __Congregational__ Allergies __NKDA_____

Admitting Diagnoses/Chief Complaint

Alzheimer's dementia

Assessment Data

G.C. is a retired architect who was just admitted to a dementia unit. His wife of 52 years has been his primary caregiver. She first noticed that something was different around 4 years ago when he started having trouble finding the word he wanted to say and didn't want to socialize with old friends or family. The disease has continued to progress to the point where his wife can no longer care for him by herself. He is often agitated and aggressive and has wandered away from home several times.

Admission assessment 1100: VS: T 37° C (98.2° F), BP 132/84, P 64 and regular, R 24 and unlabored. O$_2$ saturation 98% on RA. G.C. does not respond to questions about pain. No wincing or crying out. He is A&O to person only. PERRLA. Lungs clear. Apical is 64 and regular. Abdomen is soft with BS in all 4 quadrants. No dependent edema. Pedal pulses 2+ bilaterally. Skin is intact. Ambulates slowly, often walking in the same pattern repeatedly. G.C. responds to his name, answers questions with unrelated comments, and repeats the same questions or statements over and over. He requires assistance of 1 for dressing, bathing, toileting, oral care. His code status is DNR.

G.C.'s wife states that he usually washes in the shower, but she has had to get into the shower with him lately because he doesn't know what to do when he is in the shower alone. He needs prompts to get dressed and she helps him choose his clothes. She takes him to the bathroom every 2-3 hours when he is awake. He hasn't been eating well, so she has been trying to keep meals simple. She uses distraction and redirection when he becomes agitated. Music and television usually calm him. He likes to listen to oldies from the 50s and 60s and watches game shows on TV. He has been incontinent of urine a couple of times when they were away from home too long.

Lab Values/Diagnostic Test Results

BMP

CBC

Misc Lab Values/Diagnostic Test Results

Treatments

I&O
Fall precautions
Weekly VS
Toileting q 2 hr
Assistance with ADLs

Primary Nursing Diagnosis	Nursing Diagnosis 2	Nursing Diagnosis 3
Supporting Data	Supporting Data	Supporting Data
STG/NOC	STG/NOC	STG/NOC
Interventions/NIC with Rationale	Interventions/NIC with Rationale	Interventions/NIC with Rationale
Rationale Citation/EBP	Rationale Citation/EBP	Rationale Citation/EBP
Evaluation	Evaluation	Evaluation

ⓔAn interactive version of the Conceptual Care Map is on Evolve.

CASE STUDY

6

Danielle Hammond

Name/s _____ Date _____

Patient Assignment

D.H. is a 32-year-old female who came into the emergency department (ED) after a fall while ice skating. She states that when she fell she must have extended her right arm to break the fall because she hurt her right arm. She has a displaced, closed fracture of the right radius. She had an open reduction internal fixation (ORIF) of her right radius 2 hours ago, and has just been admitted to the orthopedic unit.

Report at 1640 from the postanesthesia case unit (PACU) nurse: Patient is stable after general anesthesia, and is allergic to penicillin (PCN). VS: T 37.5° C (99.5° F), BP 122/70, P 78 and regular, R 20 and shallow. O_2 saturation 96% on RA. A&O to person, place, and situation. PERRLA. Answering questions appropriately but sleeping intermittently. Lungs clear. Abdomen soft and nontender with hypoactive BS in all four quadrants. Voided 200 mL clear amber urine. Pedal pulses 2+. Radial pulse 2+ on left. Unable to palpate right radial pulse because of placement of a surgical splint below the elbow to the middle of the hand. Patient was given 4 mg morphine IV in the PACU at 1600 for a pain level of 8/10. States pain level is now 5/10.

Admission Orders

Admit to the orthopedic unit: Up ad lib. Vital signs q 2 hr × 2, then q 4 hr. I&O. Neurovascular checks of right hand q 2 hr. Saline lock. Flush with 10 mL NS q 8 hr. Clear liquid diet, advance as tolerated. Morphine 2 mg IV q 2 hr PRN for moderate (4-7/10) to severe (8-10/10) pain. Tramadol 100 mg PO q 6 hr PRN for moderate (4-7/10) to moderately severe (7-8/10) pain. Acetaminophen 500 mg 2 tablets PO q 6 hr PRN for mild (1-3/10) to moderate (4-7/10) pain. Docusate 100 mg PO q 12 hr. Ice to right wrist. CBC and BMP in the morning.

1. List at least four postoperative complications that are risks for D.H.

2. What are neurovascular checks?

3. What is the rationale behind ordering three different types of pain medications for D.H.? What is the classification of each?

4. As you enter D.H.'s room, what are your priority assessments?

5. What assessment findings might indicate postoperative hemorrhage?

ASSESSMENT UPDATE

1700: VS: T 36.7° C (98° F), BP 120/72, P 76 and regular, R 22 and unlabored. Pain 5/10 in right wrist and hand, dull and throbbing. Height 170.2 cm (67 in), weight 60 kg (132 lb). A&Ox4. Patient is talking to her husband who is at bedside. PERRLA. Apical pulse 76 and regular. Lungs clear. Abdomen soft with BS present in all 4 quadrants. MAE. Splint on right lower arm dry and intact. Moderate nonpitting edema of the right fingers, fingers warm, capillary refill <2 seconds. Skin warm and dry. Braden score 22. She has sensation and movement in her right fingers with no numbness or tingling. 24-gauge saline lock in left hand with no redness or swelling at insertion site. D.H states that she went ice skating this morning with her 8-year-old daughter and some friends and their children. Her daughter is with friends, and her husband was called at work when she realized she had to have surgery. She states that she has never been hurt or in the hospital before except for the birth of her daughter by uncomplicated vaginal delivery. She is right-handed and is allergic to penicillin.

6. What postoperative nursing interventions can you initiate while you assess D.H.?

7. What assessment findings would prompt you to call the surgeon?

8. List at least five nursing diagnoses or patient problems for D.H.

9. Choose three nursing diagnoses and write short-term goals for D.H.

10. Complete the CCM for Case Study 6 in this book or in the CCM Creator on Evolve for D.H. for the first evening of her hospitalization when she is first admitted to the orthopedic unit. Be sure to enter all of the data for D.H. and include classifications and rationales for medications. Cluster the data to support nursing diagnoses or patient problems, and color code the data to match the nursing diagnoses. Use the nursing diagnoses statements or patient problems and short-term goals that you identified in the case study. Evaluate the plan of care based on her assessment this evening.

11. After your initial postoperative assessment, which interventions can be delegated to the UAP?

ASSESSMENT UPDATE

The next morning you are again assigned to care for D.H. Her orders remain the same except there is now an order for PT and OT consults. She last had morphine at 2300 last night and rested most of the night. She requested tramadol instead of morphine at 0700 because she would like to "see if the pain is OK without narcotics."

When you enter the room at 0800 she is sitting up in bed eating a regular breakfast. She tells you "I might lose weight because I can barely get the food to my mouth with my left hand." Her vital signs are stable; pain level 4/10 after tramadol at 0700. Her physical assessment is normal except for the slight edema in her right hand. The surgical splint is dry and intact. She has sensation in her right fingers. Capillary refill in the right fingers is <2 seconds. Her right arm is propped up on two pillows and she has an ice pack on top of the splint.

BMP results were normal. CBC: WBC 8000 cells/mm³, Hgb 11 g/dL, Hct 35%, Platelets 200,000 cells/mm³. Lab results may vary by facility.

12. Which lab results are abnormal? What could have caused the abnormal lab results?

13. Which professional from the interdisciplinary team might the nurse consider collaborating with to help D.H. increase the oxygen carrying ability of her blood?

14. Discuss the information the nurse should provide for D.H. regarding the consult with PT.

15. Discuss patient education the nurse should provide to D.H. about the role of OT in her plan of care.

16. In anticipation for discharge, what teaching plan should be developed for D.H.? Include teaching regarding splint care, pain management, and activity level in the care plan.

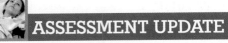

ASSESSMENT UPDATE

D.H. is being discharged in the afternoon after her consultations with dietary, OT, and PT. She dressed herself in warm-up pants and a buttoned shirt that her husband brought from home. She has rated her pain this shift at 2-3/10 and had doses of acetaminophen at 1200 for pain of 3/10. She rated the pain at 2/10 30 minutes after the acetaminophen. Her right hand is warm and slightly edematous. She has sensation in her right hand, with no numbness, tingling, or itching. Her capillary refill is <2 seconds.

17. Evaluate the plan of care again using the assessment updates for the day of discharge. Include an evaluation for each of the nursing diagnoses or patient problems.

Evaluation	Evaluation	Evaluation

Medications

Morphine 2 mg IV q 2 hr PRN for moderate to severe pain.

Tramadol 100 PO q 6 hr PRN for moderately severe pain.

Acetaminphen 500 mg 2 tablets PO q 6 hr PRN for mild pain.

Docusate 100 mg PO q 12 hr.

Conceptual Care Map

Student Name_____

Patient Initials __D.H.__ Room # _____ Admission Date _____

CODE Status _____ Today's Date _____ Age _32_ Gender _F_

Weight ___60 kg (132 lb)___ Height __170.2 cm (67 in)___

Braden Score___22___ Diet _Clear liquids, advance as tolerated_

Activity __Up ad lib__ Religion _____ Allergies ___Penicillin__

Lab Values/Diagnostic Test Results

BMP

CBC

Admitting Diagnoses/Chief Complaint

Displaced closed fracture right radius/fell skating and hurt right arm

Assessment Data

ORIF of right radius 2 hours ago, admitted to the orthopedic unit.

Report from PACU nurse 1640: Patient is stable after general anesthesia. VS: T 37.5° C (99.5° F), BP 122/70, P 78 and regular, R 20 and shallow. O₂ saturation 96% on RA. A&O to person, place and situation. PERRLA. Answering questions appropriately but sleeping intermittently. Lungs clear. Abdomen soft and nontender with hypoactive BS in all 4 quadrants. Voided 200 mL clear amber urine. Pedal pulses 2+. Radial pulse 2+ on left. Unable to palpate right radial pulse due to placement of a surgical splint below the elbow to the middle of the hand. Patient had 4 mg morphine IV in the PACU at 1600.

1700: VS: T 36.7° C (98° F), BP 120/72, P 76 and regular, R 22 and unlabored. Pain 5/10 in right wrist and hand, dull and throbbing. A&Ox4. PERRLA. Apical pulse 76 and regular. Lungs clear. Abdomen soft with BS present in all 4 quadrants. MAE. Splint on right lower arm dry and intact. Moderate nonpitting edema of the right fingers, fingers warm, capillary refill <2 seconds. Has sensation and movement in her right fingers with no numbness or tingling. Saline lock in left hand with no redness or swelling at insertion site. She is talking to her husband who is at bedside. States that she went ice skating this morning with her 8-year-old daughter and some friends and their children. States that when she fell she must have extended her right arm to break the fall because she hurt her right arm. Her daughter is with friends, and her husband was called at work when she realized she had to have surgery. She states that she has never been hurt or in the hospital before except for the birth of her daughter, by uncomplicated vaginal delivery. She is right-handed and has an allergy to penicillin.

Misc Lab Values/Diagnostic Test Results

X-ray results: right arm: displaced fracture of right radius

IV Sites/Fluids/Rate

Saline lock left hand, 24 g

Flush with 10 mL NS q 8 hr

Past Medical/Surgical History

1 pregnancy 8 years ago, uncomplicated vaginal delivery

Treatments

VS q 2 hr x 2 then q 4 hr

I&O

Neurovascular checks of right hand q2h

CBC and BMP in the morning

Ice to right wrist

Splint care

Up ad lib

Clear liquids, advance as tolerated

Primary Nursing Diagnosis	Nursing Diagnosis 2	Nursing Diagnosis 3
Supporting Data	Supporting Data	Supporting Data
STG/NOC	STG/NOC	STG/NOC
Interventions/NIC with Rationale	Interventions/NIC with Rationale	Interventions/NIC with Rationale
Rationale Citation/EBP	Rationale Citation/EBP	Rationale Citation/EBP
Evaluation	Evaluation	Evaluation

ⓔ An interactive version of the Conceptual Care Map is on Evolve.

CASE STUDY 7

Thomas Middleton

Name/s _____ **Date** _____

Patient Assignment

T.M. is a 32-year-old paraplegic male who was admitted to the medical unit 3 days ago. He was seen by his PCP in the office for a complaint of an open area on his buttock. He first noticed drainage on his underwear and asked his wife to look at the area. She noted an open sore and covered it with gauze. An appointment was made for T.M. to see his PCP. The PCP sent him to the hospital as a direct admission for treatment of a pressure injury on his right buttocks.

1. This is your first time caring for T.M. As you review the electronic health record (EHR) and gather a health history, what information will be helpful for you to know before you begin care?

2. What focused assessments will you perform during your first encounter with T.M.?

ASSESSMENT UPDATE

As you review T.M.'s EHR, you discover that he suffered a spinal cord injury at the level of T12-L1 in a motorcycle accident 3 years ago. He has paralysis of his lower extremities, loss of sensation from below his waist to his feet. He also fractured his left lower leg in the accident and had an ORIF to stabilize the fracture.

T.M. is married and has two children, ages 5 and 8. He does computer work from home, so he spends most of the day sitting in his wheelchair at a desk. His wife works outside the home as a teacher aid, so she and the children are gone during the day. The family lives in a three-bedroom ranch-style home, which has been adapted for T.M.'s wheelchair. He is able to care for himself at home and can transfer from bed to wheelchair to toilet or shower chair using his upper body. His religion is Catholic. T.M. is on an adult regular diet and has no known drug allergies. He is a full code.

Labs: BMP normal, CBC normal, serum prealbumin 14 mg/dL (Lab results may vary by facility.)

Wound culture results: negative

Current orders include: Bedrest, turn q 2 hr. Pressure-reducing mattress. DC IV ampicillin. Enoxaparin 40 mg daily subcutaneously. Dressing change: cleanse wound on right buttocks with sterile normal saline solution, apply hydrocolloid dressing. Change q 3 days, or when soiled. Physical therapy, social service, and dietary consults. I&O. Daily weights. SCDs.

3. What is a pressure injury? How do pressure injuries form?

4. List the risk factors that may have contributed to T.M.'s pressure injury.

5. What is the rationale behind T.M.'s current orders?

6. Interpret T.M.'s lab results.

7. Describe the step-by-step procedure for changing T.M.'s dressing.

ASSESSMENT UPDATE

Day 3 0830: VS: T 36.8° C (98.2° F), BP 126/68, P 64 and regular, R 20 and unlabored. O₂ saturation 96%
on RA. Denies pain. T.M. is A&Ox4, PERRLA. Lungs clear. Apical pulse is 64 and regular. Abdomen is soft and
nontender. BS present in all four quadrants. Skin warm and dry. Braden score 16. Wound on right buttocks 3.2
cm × 2.8 cm × 1 cm deep. Wound bed is red with moderate amount of exudate. No tunneling or undermining.
Wound cleansed with sterile NS. New hydrocolloid dressing applied. Pedal pulses 2+ bilaterally. SCDs in place on
both legs. 4" healed scar on the front of the left shin, which T.M. states is from the surgery following the accident.
Lower extremities are flaccid. Unable to feel sharp or dull objects touching his legs.

Weight 64.5 kg (142 lb). Height 180.3 cm (71 in). Patient states "I watch what I eat because I don't want to
get too heavy to lift myself during transfers."

T.M. states, "I feel sad that this has happened to me. I struggled after the accident, but I was finally doing well,
working hard strengthening my upper body, mostly taking care of myself, and working from home." His wife helps
him with some of his care and does ROM exercises on his legs every night before they go to sleep. T.M. says that
his wife is very supportive and has visited in the evenings while he has been in the hospital. Her parents live
nearby and help with childcare when needed.

8. According to the 2016 guidelines from the National Pressure Ulcer Advisory Panel (NPUAP), what stage of pressure injury is T.M.'s wound (National Pressure Ulcer Advisory Panel [NPUAP], April 2016. www.npuap.org/national-pressure-ulcer-advisory-panel-npuap-announces-a-change-in-terminology-from-pressure-ulcer-to-pressure-injury-and-updates-the-stages-of-pressure-injury/?platform=hootsuite.)?

9. Label each photo and describe the stage of pressure injury pictured.

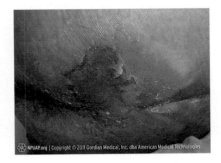

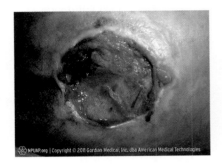

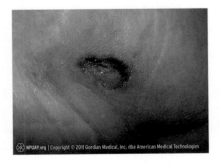

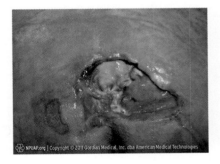

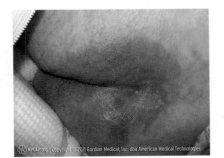

10. What is a Braden scale and what does a score of 16 mean?

11. How will T.M.'s wound most likely heal?

12. What communication techniques can you use to provide emotional support for T.M.?

13. Write a priority nursing diagnosis with diagnostic statement or patient problem for T.M.

14. Write a patient-centered, measurable goal for the priority nursing diagnosis or patient problem.

15. Begin completing a CCM for Case Study 7 in this book or in the CCM Creator on Evolve for T.M. Complete the first page, including demographic data, medications with classifications and rationales, medical and surgical history, lab results with interpretation, treatments, and assessment data. Use the priority nursing diagnostic statement or patient problem from question 13 along with two other nursing diagnoses, and formulate a plan of care for T.M. Use the Assessment Update from day 7 to complete the evaluation section of the CCM.

Day 7 0900: T.M.'s VS remain stable and his physical exam is unchanged except wound size is decreased to 3.0 cm × 2.4 cm × 0.8 cm. Wound bed is beefy red with granulation tissue. Small amount of drainage. Wound cleansed. New hydrocolloid dressing applied. Patient states that he feels encouraged because the wound is starting to heal. Wife was present during wound care and observed. She feels she could perform wound care if it was necessary. T.M. is eating 90% of his meals and drinking a protein shake that has been fortified with vitamins and minerals twice daily. Weight 65.9 kg (145 lb). He has met with the dietitian and states that he understands which foods he should eat and which supplement he should buy.

New orders: Discharge tomorrow. Referral to community agency for in-home wound care twice weekly. Wound care: Cleanse wound on right buttocks with sterile saline solution, apply hydrocolloid dressing twice weekly or when loose or soiled. Follow up with PCP in 1 week for evaluation of wound and repeat prealbumin level. Diet: high in protein, continue drinking two supplemental shakes per day. Avoid sitting on buttocks. Change positions frequently, at least every 2 hours. Gel pad for wheelchair. Pressure-reducing mattress topper.

16. When planning for T.M.'s discharge, what instructions will you give him?

Medications

Enoxaparin 40 mg daily subcut.

IV Sites/Fluids/Rate

DC IV ampicillin.

Past Medical/Surgical History

Spinal cord injury at the level of T12-L1 in a motorcycle accident 3 years ago.
Paralysis of lower extremities.
Loss of sensation below the waist.
ORIF fractured left lower leg 3 years ago.

Conceptual Care Map

Student Name_____

Patient Initials __T.M.__ Room # _____ Admission Date _3 days ago_

CODE Status __Full__ Today's Date _____ Age _32_ Gender _M_

Weight __64.5 kg (142 lb)__ Height __180.3 cm (71 in)__

Braden Score _16_ Diet __Adult regular__ Activity _____ bed rest

Religion _____Catholic_____ Allergies _____NKDA_____

Admitting Diagnoses/Chief Complaint

Pressure injury right buttocks/Open area on right buttocks with drainage

Assessment Data

T.M. is paraplegic. First noticed drainage on his underwear and asked his wife to look at the area. She noted an open sore and covered it with gauze. An appointment was made for T.M. to see his PCP. Seen by his PCP in the office for a complaint of an open area on his buttock. The PCP sent him to the hospital as a direct admission.

T.M. is married and has two children, ages 5 and 8. He does computer work from home, so he spends most of the day sitting in his wheelchair at a desk. His wife works outside the home as a teacher aid, so she and the children are gone during the day. The family lives in a three-bedroom ranch-style home, which has been adapted for T.M.'s wheelchair. He is able to care for himself at home and can transfer from bed to wheelchair to toilet or shower chair using his upper body.

Day 3: VS: T 36.8° C (98.2° F), BP 126/68, P 64 and regular, R 20 and unlabored. O_2 saturation 96% on RA. Denies pain. T.M. is A&Ox4, PERRLA. Lungs clear. Apical pulse is 64 and regular. Abdomen is soft and nontender. BS present in all four quadrants. Skin warm and dry. Wound on right buttocks 3.2 cm x 2.8 cm x 1 cm deep. Wound bed is red with moderate amount of exudate. No tunneling or undermining. Pedal pulses 2+ bilaterally. SCDs in place on both legs. 4" healed scar on the front of the left shin, which T.M. states is from the surgery following the accident. Lower extremities are flaccid. Unable to feel sharp or dull objects touching his legs. Patient states, "I watch what I eat because I don't want to get too heavy to lift myself during transfers."

T.M. states, "I feel sad that this has happened to me." He states, "I struggled after the accident, but I was finally doing well, working hard strengthening my upper body, mostly taking care of myself, and working from home." His wife helps him some with his care and does ROM exercises on his legs every night before they go to sleep. T.M. says that his wife is very supportive and has visited in the evenings while he has been in the hospital. Her parents live nearby and help with childcare when needed.

Lab Values/Diagnostic Test Results

BMP: normal

CBC: normal

Misc Lab Values/Diagnostic Test Results

Serum prealbumin 14 mg/dL
Wound culture: negative

Treatments

Bed rest
Turn q 2 hr
Pressure-reducing mattress
Cleanse wound on right buttocks with sterile normal saline solution, apply hydrocolloidal dressing. Change q 3 days, or when soiled.
Physical therapy
Social service
Dietary consult
I&O
Daily weights
SCDs

Primary Nursing Diagnosis	Nursing Diagnosis 2	Nursing Diagnosis 3
Supporting Data	Supporting Data	Supporting Data
STG/NOC	STG/NOC	STG/NOC
Interventions/NIC with Rationale	Interventions/NIC with Rationale	Interventions/NIC with Rationale
Rationale Citation/EBP	Rationale Citation/EBP	Rationale Citation/EBP
Evaluation	Evaluation	Evaluation

ⓔ An interactive version of the Conceptual Care Map is on Evolve.

CASE STUDY 8

Beatrice Keifer

Name/s _____ Date _____

Patient Assignment

B.K. is an 82-year-old Caucasian female who was admitted to the hospital with compression fractures of L1 and L2. She presented to the emergency department (ED) with severe pain in her back that she rated 8/10. Her medical and surgical history shows that she was diagnosed with osteopenia in her hips and spine at age 64 and had a total hysterectomy at age 62. Height 162.6 cm (64 in), weight 56.4 kg (124 lb). B.K. has remained active, goes to walk aerobics classes five times per week; modified her diet to include calcium-rich foods; and took calcium supplements and a multivitamin. She states that she was in aerobics class exercising as usual when she felt a sudden sharp pain in her back. She is married and has three grown children and seven grandchildren who all live within 30 minutes of her. Her husband is at her bedside.

CBC, BMP, Ca, vitamin D level, and CT scan of the spine were done on admission. All lab and diagnostic tests were normal except: Ca 8 mg/dL, vitamin D 16 pg/dL, and CT of the spine showed uncomplicated compression fractures of L1 and L2.

Admission Orders

Vital signs q 4 hr with O_2 sat, saline lock, I&O, adult regular diet, up ad lib, avoid twisting at the waist. Dual-energy x-ray absorptiometry (DEXAscan). Hydrocodone 5 mg/acetaminophen 325 mg, one tablet q 6 hr PO PRN for pain. Docusate 100 mg, one tablet PO q 12 hr. Enoxaparin 40 mg daily subcutaneously. SCDs while in bed.

1. Identify the risk factors that could have contributed to B.K.'s fractures.

2. How are B.K.'s lab values related to her spinal fractures?

3. What is the purpose of ordering docusate?

4. What positive lifestyle changes did B.K. make when she found out she had osteopenia?

5. What are your assessment priorities as you begin to care for B.K.?

6. List some assessment questions that you will ask during your first encounter with B.K.

ASSESSMENT UPDATE

As the nurse taking care of B.K. your initial assessment findings at 0800 include: VS: T 36.8° C (98.2° F), BP 122/64, P 84 and regular, R 24 and unlabored. O$_2$ saturation 95% on RA. Pain level 7/10 in the lower back, it is sharp and constant and does not radiate to her legs. The pain intensifies to 9/10 with movement. B.K. is A&Ox4. PERRLA. Lungs are clear. Apical pulse is 84 and regular. Abdomen is soft and nontender, with bowel sounds (BS) present in all four quadrants. Sensation in lower extremities is normal and pedal pulses are 2+. No edema in legs or feet. Skin warm and dry with no lesions. Saline lock with 22 g IV catheter in left wrist without redness or swelling. B.K. states that she has been up to the bathroom twice during the night with her husband's help. MAE. She states it is difficult to get her legs over to the edge of the bed so she isn't moving much, and that when she first stands, it "hurts a lot."

B.K. is Protestant, has allergies to shellfish and bee stings, and is a full code.

7. List at least three nursing diagnoses or problems for this patient, with "related to" statements and supporting data or risk factors.

8. Write a short-term goal for each of the nursing diagnoses in question 7.

9. List some interventions that are important as you begin to care for B.K.

ASSESSMENT UPDATE

B.K. went to the Radiology Department and had a DEXAscan. The results show a T score of -2.9 in her spine and -2.4 in her hips. A T score of -1.0 to -2.5 indicates osteopenia and a T score of >2.5 indicates osteoporosis. B.K. has osteopenia in her hips and osteoporosis in her spine.

10. What classifications of medication would you anticipate being recommended to B.K. by her primary care provider (PCP) since she has been diagnosed with osteoporosis?

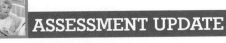

ASSESSMENT UPDATE

On the second morning, the night nurse reports that B.K. slept at short intervals but is still experiencing pain of 7/10 when she ambulates to the bathroom, even after being medicated for pain. When you walk into her room at 0745 B.K. is awake and eating breakfast. She states that she doesn't have much of an appetite but is drinking a lot of water and juice. Her vital signs are stable except that she rates her pain at 6/10 while sitting in bed and her physical exam is unchanged. She states that the pain is intense when she ambulates. She last had pain medication at 0300. She states she has not had a bowel movement since admission, but she hasn't eaten very much.

11. What complementary and alternative pain management techniques might be used with B.K.? Which of these would require collaboration with the PCP?

12. What interventions will help B.K. have a bowel movement?

13. Complete the CCM for Case Study 8 in this book or in the CCM Creator on Evolve for B.K. for the second morning of her hospitalization. Add the medication classifications and rationales, and interpret the lab values in the data collection portion of the CCM. Prioritize the nursing diagnoses statements and short-term goals that you identified in the case study by clustering the data, and write an individualized plan of care for B.K. Use the Assessment Updates that follow to evaluate the care plan.

ASSESSMENT UPDATE

When you give report at 1900 to the next shift, you tell the night nurse that during your 12-hour shift B.K. has been using deep breathing exercises and listening to classical music to complement her pain medication. She ambulates slowly in her room and in the hallway with her husband by her side. B.K. was still reporting pain of 6/10 while in bed and 7/10 when moving. After discussing B.K.'s pain level with the PCP, new orders at 1600 include: ibuprofen 400 mg PO q 8 hr PRN for mild to moderate pain, heat applied to lumbar area with aquathermia pad for 20 minutes q 3 hr PRN. She has had one dose of ibuprofen 4 hours after her last dose of hydrocodone/acetaminophen, and one heat treatment. She reported her pain at a level of 3/10 when sitting in bed after her treatment.

B.K. had a soft, brown, formed bowel movement at 1400. She consumed 75% of her lunch, 50% of her dinner, and drank 1500 mL of fluid during the shift. B.K. states that her "stomach feels less bloated." Abdomen soft and nontender. BS present in all four quadrants.

14. Rewrite your report to the night nurse in an SBAR handoff format.

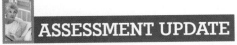

ASSESSMENT UPDATE

The next morning when you report for your shift, the night nurse tells you that B.K. had a good night and that there is an order for her discharge. Her pain has been 3-5/10 during the night, and she slept two long intervals. The PCP wrote a new prescription for B.K. for ibandronate 150 mg once monthly.

15. What discharge instructions will be important for B.K.?

Medications

Hydrocodone 5 mg/acetaminophen 325 mg, one tablet PO q 6 hr for pain.
Docusate 100 mg, one tablet PO q 12 hr.
Enoxaparin 40 mg daily subcut.

IV Sites/Fluids/Rate

Saline lock 22 g in left wrist, no redness or swelling

Past Medical/Surgical History

Total hysterectomy age 64

Osteopenia age 62

Takes calcium supplements and a multivitamin

Conceptual Care Map

Student Name_____

Patient Initials _B.K._ Room #_____ Admission Date_____

CODE Status __Full__ Today's Date_____ Age_82_ Gender _F_

Weight _56.4 kg (124 lb)_ Height _162.6 cm (64 in)_

Braden Score _21_ Diet _Adult regular_ Activity _Up ad lib, avoid twisting at the waist_ Religion _Protestant_ Allergies _Shellfish, bee stings_

Admitting Diagnoses/Chief Complaint

Compression fractures L1, L2/severe pain 8/10 in back

Assessment Data

B.K. is an 82 year old female admitted with compression fractures of L1 and L2. She presented to the ED with severe pain in her back that she rated 8/10. She has remained active, goes to walk aerobics classes five times per week; follows diet of calcium-rich foods. States she was in aerobics class exercising and felt a sudden sharp pain in her back. Married with three grown children and seven grandchildren, all live within 30 minutes of her. Husband is at bedside.

0800 VS: T 36.8° C (98.2° F), BP 122/64, P 84 and regular, R 24 and unlabored. O_2 95% on RA. Pain 7/10 in the lower back, sharp and constant, does not radiate to her legs, intensifies to 9/10 with movement. A&Ox4. PERRLA. Lungs clear. Apical pulse is 84 and regular. Abdomen soft and nontender BS present in all four quadrants. Sensation in lower extremities is normal and pedal pulses are 2+. No edema in legs or feet. Skin is warm and dry with no lesions. States she has been up to the bathroom twice during the night with her husband's help. MAE. She states it is difficult to get her legs over to the edge of the bed, so she isn't moving much; when she first stands, it "hurts a lot."

Day 2 morning report: slept at short intervals, pain of 7/10 when ambulating to the bathroom, even after being medicated for pain. 0745: awake and eating breakfast. States she doesn't have much of an appetite but is drinking a lot of water and juice. VS stable except pain at 6/10 while sitting in bed, and "intense" when she ambulates. Physical exam unchanged. Last pain medication at 0300. No bowel movement since admission, but she hasn't eaten very much.

Lab Values/Diagnostic Test Results

BMP: normal

CBC: normal

Misc Lab Values/Diagnostic Test Results

Test Results

Vitamin D 16 pg/dL ↓

Calcium 8 mg/dL ↓

CT scan of spine: uncomplicated compression fractures of L1, L2

DEXAscan: pending

Treatments

VS q 4 hr with O_2 sat

I&O

Up ad lib, avoid twisting at the waist

Adult regular diet

CBC

BMP

DEXAscan: pending

SCDs while in bed

Primary Nursing Diagnosis	Nursing Diagnosis 2	Nursing Diagnosis 3
Supporting Data	Supporting Data	Supporting Data
STG/NOC	STG/NOC	STG/NOC
Interventions/NIC with Rationale	Interventions/NIC with Rationale	Interventions/NIC with Rationale
Rationale Citation/EBP	Rationale Citation/EBP	Rationale Citation/EBP
Evaluation	Evaluation	Evaluation

ⓔ An interactive version of the Conceptual Care Map is on Evolve.

CASE STUDY

9

Vera Rose

Name/s _____ Date _____

Patient Assignment

V.R. is a 55-year-old female admitted to the hospital 10 days ago with shortness of breath, fever, vomiting, and nausea. She was diagnosed with community-acquired pneumonia 2 days before admission and given a prescription for oral antibiotics from her primary care provider (PCP). She began vomiting and could not keep anything down, and her respiratory symptoms worsened, so she came to the emergency department (ED). After being hospitalized, she received a 10-day course of levofloxacin 500 mg IV qd. She began having diarrhea, several times each day, 2 days ago. A stool culture was sent and is positive for *Clostridium difficile* (*C. difficile* or C-diff). V.R. is now having watery diarrhea six to eight times per day associated with abdominal cramping, nausea, and urgency. She has lost 2.3 kg (5 lb) in the past 3 days and has been running a low fever. She is allergic to penicillin (PCN) and is a full code.

Current Orders

IV fluids D_5 0.45% NS 75 mL/hr. DC levofloxacin. Enoxaparin 40 mg daily subcutaneously. SCDs while in bed. Up ad lib. VS q 4 hr. Metronidazole 500 mg/100 mL premixed injectable solution IV q 8 hr, infuse over 60 minutes. Contact precautions. Clear liquid diet, advance as tolerated. BMP & CBC in the morning. I&O. Daily weight.

1. What is C-diff and how is it spread?

2. What risk factors did V.R. have for developing C-diff?

3. What are contact precautions?

4. Identify the classification and the purpose of the current medications that are ordered for V.R. Add these medications to the data collection portion of the CCM.

5. What abnormal lab values would you anticipate when her CBC and BMP are drawn tomorrow?

ASSESSMENT UPDATE

Day 11 0830: VS: T 38.2° C (100.8° F), BP 106/60, P 82 and regular, R 24 and unlabored. O_2 saturation 94% on RA. Pain level at 6/10 when she has abdominal cramping. She is A&Ox4, PERRLA. Lungs clear. Apical pulse is 82 and regular. Abdomen is firm and tender with hyperactive BS in all four quadrants. Skin warm and dry. Pedal pulses 2+ bilaterally. Musculoskeletal assessment is normal. SCDs in place on both legs. Height 167.6 cm (66 in). Weight 73.2 kg (161 lb). She has redness and excoriation of her perianal area. Braden score 18. Her IV fluids are running in a 22-gauge IV catheter in her right hand, and she has a 24-gauge saline lock in her left forearm. Both IV sites are without redness or swelling.

V.R. states that she is so weak she can barely get to the bathroom by herself. A couple of times she "almost didn't make it to the bathroom on time." She states that she has had diarrhea three times already since she woke up this morning, and it is "watery and it smells." She naps several times a day. She is "tired of being in this hospital and feels so alone." Her children were visiting and were at the hospital 3 days ago, but she does not want them to visit now because they "might catch something." She told the pastor at her United Methodist Church not to come and visit for the same reason. V.R. is divorced, and her adult daughter lives with her. She has a son who is married, lives nearby, and has a 1-year-old daughter. V.R. works as an administrative assistant. She states, "I am concerned because I am missing so much work. I am almost out of sick days and will have to start using vacation days to keep getting paid."

Lab results: BMP: sodium 146 mEq/L; potassium 4.0; chloride 105 mEq/L; bicarbonate 22 mEq/L; BUN 22 mg/dL; creatinine 1.3 mg/dL; glucose 80 mg/dL

CBC: hemoglobin 16 g/dL; hematocrit 49%; white blood cells 12,000 mm³; platelets 250,000 mm³

Lab results may vary by facility.

6. Which assessment and lab findings are abnormal? What would be the normal findings? Give a rationale for the abnormal lab values. Add the lab values and interpret the meaning of any abnormal values in lab results section of the CCM.

7. How will you explain the current orders to V.R.?

8. Based on your current assessment findings, identify your highest-priority nursing diagnosis with statement or patient problem, for V.R. What is the rationale behind choosing this diagnosis?

9. Write a patient goal statement for your priority nursing diagnosis or patient problem.

10. List at least two other nursing diagnoses or patient problems for V.R.

11. Complete a CCM for Case Study 9 in this book or in the CCM Creator on Evolve for V.R. Choose two nursing diagnoses labels or patient problems from question 10 in addition to the priority nursing diagnosis listed in question 8. Write short-term goals for each problem and interventions designed to help the patient reach the goals. Remember to use EBP citations for each intervention's rationale, and include your evaluation based on how V.R. responds to the interventions by day 14 of her hospitalization.

12. What are some nursing interventions that are important for V.R.? List at least five.

13. Three days after V.R. started on IV metronidazole, you are again assigned to care for her. What are your priority assessments based on previous findings?

ASSESSMENT UPDATE

Day 14, 0900 VS: T 36.8° C (98.2° F), BP 118/70, P 68 and regular, R 20 and unlabored. O$_2$ saturation 96% on RA. Pain level 0/10. She is having no abdominal cramping. She is A&O×4, PERRLA. Lungs clear. Apical pulse is 68 and regular. Abdomen is soft and slightly tender with normal BS in all four quadrants. Skin warm and dry. Pedal pulses 2+ bilaterally. SCDs in place on both legs when patient is in bed. Weight 74.1 kg (163 lb). Slight redness of her perianal area. Braden score 20. 22-gauge saline lock in her right forearm is without redness or swelling. Repeat stool cultures were obtained yesterday and results are pending.

V.R. is eating 75% of meals and drinking 1500 mL of fluids each day. She is still on metronidazole IV through her saline lock but the IV fluids were discontinued yesterday. Intake yesterday = 1800 mL. Output = 1600 mL urine, three soft formed stools. V.R. is up in her room most of the day either walking or sitting in the chair. She states that she still feels "tired but is starting to feel better." She says that she "misses her children and grand-daughter and can't wait to get home."

New orders: Discharge tomorrow pending results from repeat stool cultures. Metronidazole 500 mg PO q 8 hr × 7 days. Follow up with PCP in 1 week. Do not return to work until after follow-up appointment with PCP. Diet as tolerated.

14. When planning for V.R.'s discharge, what instructions will you give her?

Medications

Enoxaparin 40 mg subcut daily

~~Levofloxacin 500 mg IV qd. X 10 days~~
DCd

Metronidazole 500 mg/100 mL premixed injectable solution IV q 8 hr, infuse over 60 minutes

IV Sites/Fluids/Rate

D5 0.45% NS 75 mL/hr in right hand 22-g IV catheter
Saline lock left forearm, 24-g catheter

Past Medical/Surgical History

Community-acquired pneumonia

Conceptual Care Map

Student Name_____
Patient Initials _V.R._ Room # _____ Admission Date _10 days ago_
CODE Status _Full_ Today's Date _____ Age _55_ Gender _F_
Weight _73.2 kg (161 lb)_ Height _167.6 cm (66 in)_
Braden Score _18_ Diet _Clear liquids, advance as tolerated_
Activity _Up ad lib_ Religion _United Methodist_ Allergies _PCN_

Admitting Diagnoses/Chief Complaint

Community-acquired pneumonia/shortness of breath, fever, vomiting, nausea

Assessment Data

Diagnosed with community-acquired pneumonia 2 days before admission and given a prescription for oral antibiotics from her PCP. She began vomiting and couldn't keep anything down, respiratory symptoms worsened. After being hospitalized, she received a 10-day course of levofloxacin. She began having diarrhea several times each day 2 days ago. A stool culture was sent and is positive for *Clostridium difficile* (*C. difficile* or C-diff). V.R. is now having watery diarrhea six to eight times per day associated with abdominal cramping, nausea, and urgency. She has lost 2.3 kg (5 lb) in the past 3 days and has been running a low fever.

0830: VS: T 38.2° C (100.8° F), BP 106/60, P 82 and regular, R 24 and unlabored. O₂ saturation 94% on RA. Pain level at 6/10 when she has abdominal cramping. She is A&O×4, PERRLA. Lungs clear. Apical pulse 82 and regular. Abdomen is firm and tender with hyperactive BS in all four quadrants. Skin warm and dry. Pedal pulses 2+ bilaterally. Musculoskeletal assessment normal. SCDs in place on both legs. Weight 161 lb. She has redness and excoriation of her perianal area. Both IV sites are without redness or swelling.

V.R. states that she is so weak that she can barely get to the bathroom by herself. A couple of times she "almost didn't make it to the bathroom on time." She states that she has had diarrhea three times already since she woke up this morning, and it is "watery and it smells." She naps several times a day. She is "tired of being in this hospital and feels so alone." Her children were visiting and were at the hospital 3 days ago, but she doesn't want them to visit now because they "might catch something." She told the pastor at her United Methodist Church not to come and visit. V.R. is divorced, and her adult daughter lives with her. She also has a son who is married, lives nearby, and has a 1-year-old daughter. V.R. works as an administrative assistant. She states "I am concerned because I am missing so much work. I am almost out of sick days and will have to start using vacation days in order to keep getting paid."

Lab Values/Diagnostic Test Results

BMP

CBC

Misc Lab Values/Diagnostic Test Results

CBC & BMP pending
Stool culture: positive for *Clostridium difficile*

Treatments

SCDs
Up ad lib
Clear liquids, advance as tolerated
BMP & CBC in am
Contact precautions
VS q 4 hr
I&O
Daily weight
Barrier cream to perianal area after cleansing

Primary Nursing Diagnosis	Nursing Diagnosis 2	Nursing Diagnosis 3
Supporting Data	**Supporting Data**	**Supporting Data**
STG/NOC	**STG/NOC**	**STG/NOC**
Interventions/NIC with Rationale	**Interventions/NIC with Rationale**	**Interventions/NIC with Rationale**
Rationale Citation/EBP	**Rationale Citation/EBP**	**Rationale Citation/EBP**
Evaluation	**Evaluation**	**Evaluation**

ⓔ An interactive version of the Conceptual Care Map is on Evolve.

CASE STUDY 10

Cora Jenkins

Name/s _____ Date _____

Patient Assignment

C.J. is a 71-year-old female who presented to the emergency department (ED) 6 hours ago with nausea, hematemesis, and epigastric pain. She was admitted to the hospital with a diagnosis of acute GI bleed, and made NPO. A 16-g intracath was placed in her left forearm. 1000 mL of 0.9 NS was initiated at 100 mL/hr per primary care provider (PCP) order. An NG tube was placed and attached to intermittent low wall suction. 400 mL of red-tinged drainage was visible in the NG collection container within 30 minutes of insertion. She has had one melena stool since her admission. C.J. is a full code with an allergy to penicillin (PCN) and a Braden score of 20.

Initial Assessment

Upon arrival on the medical surgical unit, VS: T 37.5° C (98.6° F), BP 106/54, P 114 and regular, R 22 and shallow. O_2 saturation is 96% on RA. C.J. reports a pain level of 6/10 in her epigastric area that is cramping and intermittent, "coming in waves." C.J. is A&O×4, PERRLA, apical pulse is rapid and steady at 114. Lung sounds are clear bilaterally; her abdomen is soft, extremely tender on light palpation with rebound tenderness and hyperactive bowel sounds in the LUQ, RUQ, and LLQ, and normal in the RLQ. Occasional borborygmi are present. MAE. Dorsalis pedis pulses are 2+ bilaterally without any dependent edema present. C.J. states, "I have been nauseated occasionally for the last few weeks on and off. Then this morning I started having severe cramping and vomiting that wouldn't stop. I decided to come into the emergency room when I noticed the blood and the pain got too bad." IV site: LFA 16 g without redness, tenderness, or swelling; transparent dressing in place, signed and dated. 1000 mL 0.9 NS running at 100 mL/hr on infusion pump.

1. List a minimum of three pieces of objective data from the initial assessment that support C.J.'s admitting diagnosis of acute GI bleed.

2. Define the terms hematemesis, coffee-ground emesis, hematochezia, and melena. Briefly explain when each one might be present in a GI bleed.

3. C.J.'s basic demographic data and some ED-related treatments have been entered into the CCM. Continue filling out the demographic data and assessment areas of the CCM for Case Study 10 in this book or in the CCM Creator on Evolve.

4. Identify a minimum of three underlying etiologies for upper GI bleed.

5. Write a minimum of seven assessment questions that you as the nurse need to ask C.J. during her admission interview on the medical-surgical unit to get a better idea of what may have caused the bleeding.

6. The PCP asks you to check C.J. for orthostatic hypotension. Explain what orthostatic hypotension is and how to assess for it. What is the rationale for assessing it in C.J.?

7. During your interview and assessment of C.J., she shares that she has been taking ibuprofen 600 mg three times a day for the past 3 months because of pain in her left knee following a tennis injury. Explain the significance of this assessment finding to your understanding of C.J.'s current condition.

8. The PCP orders hydromorphone 0.2 mg/mL PCA. Demand 0.2 mg, lockout 10 minutes, 5 mg/4hr limit for C.J. Why is this medication being ordered for C.J.? What is the drug classification of Hydromorphone? What does PCA stand for and how does it work?

   a. Enter the hydromorphone order into the CCM providing its classification and rationale for administration to C.J.

9. What patient assessments should be completed before initiating a PCA infusion of hydromorphone on every patient? Provide a rationale for each assessment. Place an asterisk next to the highest-priority assessment, both before and after the PCA infusion is initiated.

10. Write two nursing diagnoses for C.J. at this point in her care, and identify short-term goals for each. Add them to your CCM care plan for C.J.

11. C.J. is scheduled for an esophagogastroduodenoscopy (EGD) in 2 hours. Briefly explain the purpose of an EGD. Provide a detailed explanation of nursing care that should be given to C.J. before her EGD, including important aspects of patient education.

12. C.J. is ordered to receive 2 to 40 mg doses of IV omeprazole in 100 mL of NS to infuse over 20 minutes each. Omeprazole is available in a vial containing 40 mg of powder and 10 mL of special solvent for reconstitution.

    a. Explain the steps required for reconstituting powdered medication for infusion.

    b. At what rate should the IV infusion pump be set to ensure that the patient receives each 40-mg dose of omeprazole in 20 minutes?

13. List essential post-EGD nursing interventions for all patients undergoing this procedure.

ASSESSMENT UPDATE

EGD results note a small tear in the mucosal lining of the stomach and the presence of H. pylori bacteria indicating the presence of peptic ulcer disease (PUD). The tear was cauterized and C.J.'s NG tube was discontinued following the procedure.

She is allowed to progress to a soft diet and oral medication and instructed to discontinue use of any NSAIDs without consultation with her PCP.

C.J. is ordered omeprazole 20 mg bid PO for 4 weeks, clarithyromycin 500 mg bid PO for 14 days, and amoxicillin 1 g bid PO for 14 days. Discharge planning within 48 hours is initiated.

14. Add the newly prescribed medications to the CCM. For each medication, note the drug classification and rationale for prescribing it for C.J.

15. Before administering C.J.'s first dose of amoxicillin, you call to clarify the order with the PCP. What is your rationale for doing this, and what is the likely outcome of your call?

16. Because C.J. was diagnosed with peptic ulcer disease, she requires nutritional guidance. A referral to what member of the health care team would be helpful in providing this information? List at least four considerations that this health care team member will share with C.J. to avoid potential exacerbation of her condition.

17. Add a third nursing diagnosis and short-term goal (STG) to your CCM based on C.J.'s new medical diagnosis of PUD. Complete the care plan for C.J. by adding interventions, rationales with citations, and evaluation statements for each of the three nursing diagnoses.

Medications

Conceptual Care Map

Student Name_____

Patient Initials __C.J.__ Room # _____ Admission Date _____

CODE Status _____ Today's Date _____

Age _71_ Gender _F_ Weight _____ Height _____ Braden Score _____

Diet _____ Activity _____

Religion _____ Allergies _____

Admitting Diagnoses/Chief Complaint
Acute GI Bleed

Lab Values/Diagnostic Test Results
BMP

CBC

Misc Lab Values/Diagnostic Test Results

Assessment Data

IV Sites/Fluids/Rate
16 g intracath LFA patent without redness or swelling, dressing dry and intact, signed and dated
1000 mL 0.9 NS @ 100 mL

Past Medical/Surgical History

Treatments
NPO
NG to intermittent low wall suction

Primary Nursing Diagnosis	Nursing Diagnosis 2	Nursing Diagnosis 3
Supporting Data	Supporting Data	Supporting Data
STG/NOC	STG/NOC	STG/NOC
Interventions/NIC with Rationale	Interventions/NIC with Rationale	Interventions/NIC with Rationale
Rationale Citation/EBP	Rationale Citation/EBP	Rationale Citation/EBP
Evaluation	Evaluation	Evaluation

ⓔ An interactive version of the Conceptual Care Map is on Evolve.

CASE STUDY 11

Helen Williams

Name/s _____   Date _____

Patient Assignment

H.W. is a 57-year-old female patient admitted to your nursing unit from the PACU following an abdominal hysterectomy. Her son and husband are with her. She is able to assist the transport team with her transfer from the cart to her bed with minimal assistance. Although she appears lethargic, H.W. is able to follow directions and answers questions appropriately when asked. Preoperative documentation indicates that H.W. is a full code. Her religious preference is Episcopal. She is 167.6 cm (66 in) tall and weighs 67.3 kg (148 lb) and currently NPO. H.W. is allergic to codeine. Her admitting diagnosis is uterine fibroids.

Initial Assessment

H.W. is A&O×4, PERRLA, with a Braden score of 20. VS: T 36.8° C (98.2° F), BP 124/76, P 70 and regular, R 18 and unlabored. O_2 saturation is 98% on RA. She reports a pain level of 4/10 across her lower abdomen, stating that the pain is "a dull ache that becomes more intense when I move." Her lungs are clear in all lobes. Her abdomen is slightly distended with hypoactive bowel sounds present in all four quadrants. She has a lower abdominal dressing placed horizontally that is dry and intact, signed and dated. An indwelling catheter is in place. H.W.'s posterior tibial pulses are 2+ bilaterally. No dependent edema noted. She has 1000 mL of D_5W at 125 mL/hr infusing into her right hand.

1. Enter H.W.'s initial assessment data into the CCM for Case Study 11 in this book or in the CCM Creator on Evolve.

2. What additional information is needed to complete the assessment documentation related to H.W.'s indwelling catheter and IV?

3. Identify a minimum of five aspects of care that you can delegate as the RN to UAP when a patient is being admitted to your nursing unit for the first time.

4. List a minimum of three actions that an RN can never delegate to a UAP during a patient's hospitalization.

5. Add each of the following postoperative orders to your CCM in the appropriate subsections. Be sure to provide classifications and rationales for each of the medications.

   Postoperative orders: VS q 4 hr, up in chair today, then up ad lib, advance diet as tolerated, morphine sulfate 2 mg IVP q 4 hr PRN, prochlorperazine 5 mg IV q 3-4 hr PRN, cough and deep breathing exercises, incentive spirometry q 1 hr while awake, sequential compression device (SCD) while in bed, DC urinary catheter, and I&O.

6. What are the expected outcomes and potential side effects of both morphine sulfate and prochlorperazine?

7. What vital sign should be monitored especially closely while a patient is taking morphine sulfate?

8. What is the antidote for morphine sulfate?

9. What additional classification of medication should be ordered for H.W. because she is taking morphine sulfate?

10. Explain the step-by-step procedure for discontinuing an indwelling urinary catheter.

11. Sometimes after a urinary catheter has been discontinued, a patient may have difficulty urinating. What are some nursing strategies that can encourage urination in patients who are having difficulty emptying their bladders?

12. What nursing intervention is best to determine the extent of urinary retention in patients experiencing bladder distention and urinary retention?

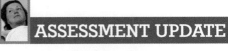

ASSESSMENT UPDATE

H.W. is unable to void 7 hours after her indwelling catheter is discontinued. She is reporting increased pain in her lower abdominal area and feeling "like I really need to go to the bathroom." Her P and BP are increased at 90 bpm and 142/82.

13. When you notify the primary care provider (PCP) that H.W. is distended and unable to urinate, an order for an indwelling catheter is written. Explain the step-by-step procedure for inserting a urinary catheter on a female patient.

14. If, on the first attempt to insert the catheter, you accidently place it into the vagina instead of the urethra, what action should you take next? Provide a rationale for your actions.

15. List a minimum of four risk factors for catheter-associated urinary tract infection (CAUTI).

16. Describe at least six procedures that should be followed to prevent CAUTI. Provide a rationale for each intervention.

ASSESSMENT UPDATE

H.W. is scheduled for discharge, however before leaving she spikes a temperature of 39° C (102.2° F). Her urine appears cloudy and slightly pink. H.W. is complaining of urgency and burning with urination. Her abdominal incision is well approximated without extreme redness, edema, or drainage. Staples are intact.

17. H.W. is diagnosed with a hospital-associated infection (HAI). What is the most likely cause of her infection?

18. What diagnostic tests would you anticipate being ordered on H.W.? Provide the normal range for each and a rationale for the PCP ordering them for H.W.

19. Develop a complete patient-centered care plan with three nursing diagnoses or patient problem statements on the CCM.

Conceptual Care Map

Medications

Student Name _____

Patient Initials __H.W.__ **Room #** _____ **Admission Date** _____

CODE Status __Full__ **Today's Date** _____ **Age** _57_ **Gender** _F_

Weight _67.3 kg (148 lb)_ **Height** _167.6 cm (66 in)_ **Braden Score** _____

Diet __NPO__ _____ **Activity** _____

_____ **Religion** ___Episcopal___ **Allergies** ___codeine___

Admitting Diagnoses/Chief Complaint
Uterine Fibroids

Lab Values/Diagnostic Test Results
BMP

CBC

Misc Lab Values/Diagnostic Test Results

Assessment Data
Admit from PACU. Appears lethargic. Able to follow directions and assist with transfer with minimal assistance.

Answers questions appropriately. Husband and son at bedside.

IV Sites/Fluids/Rate

Past Medical/Surgical History
Status post abdominal hysterectomy

Treatments

Primary Nursing Diagnosis	Nursing Diagnosis 2	Nursing Diagnosis 3
Supporting Data	Supporting Data	Supporting Data
STG/NOC	STG/NOC	STG/NOC
Interventions/NIC with Rationale	Interventions/NIC with Rationale	Interventions/NIC with Rationale
Rationale Citation/EBP	Rationale Citation/EBP	Rationale Citation/EBP
Evaluation	Evaluation	Evaluation

ⓔ An interactive version of the Conceptual Care Map is on Evolve.

CASE STUDY 12

James Robertson

Name/s _____ Date _____

Patient Assignment

J.R. is a 24-year-old male who is just being admitted to the medical unit for monitoring and medication adjustment following generalized tonic-clonic seizures at work. He has a history of epilepsy since childhood. A co-worker called 911 after J.R. "fell to the floor and began shaking." When emergency medical technicians (EMTs) arrived, the seizure had stopped. Another seizure started about 2 minutes later, so the decision was made to transport him to the emergency department (ED).

Admission Orders

Seizure precautions, VS q 4 hr, adult regular diet, I&O, saline lock, 10 mL saline flush q 8 hr, full code status, EEG this afternoon, carbamazepine 400 mg PO bid, labs: carbamazepine blood level, CBC, BMP, LFT, fasting lipid panel, and urinalysis.

1. As the admitting nurse, what focused questions should you ask J.R. about his seizure and epilepsy?

2. Which focused assessments will be important when you examine J.R.?

3. What type of seizure did J.R. have? How does this differ from other types of seizures? Describe each type of seizure.

4. What seizure precautions will the staff put into place in J.R.'s room? Give a rationale for each precaution.

5. What procedures should be followed if J.R. has another seizure?

6. What is the classification of carbamazepine?

7. What is the rationale behind the ordered lab tests: carbamazepine blood level, CBC, BMP, LFT, fasting lipid panel, and urinalysis?

ASSESSMENT UPDATE

Your initial exam of J.R. is conducted at 1400, about 3 hours after the seizures occurred: VS: T 36.2.5° C (97.2° F), BP 122/76, P 62 and regular, R 16 and unlabored. O_2 saturation 94% on RA. Height 177.8 cm (70 in). Weight 82.7 kg (182 lb). He states that his arms and legs hurt a bit; rates the pain at 2/10. A&Ox4. PERRLA. Head and neck exam is normal with no JVD. Says he still feels a bit "weird" from the seizures and correctly states the date but is unsure about the time. J.R. is answering questions appropriately and says he remembers "feeling funny" before the seizure but doesn't remember anything else until he was in the ambulance. 20-gauge saline lock in left forearm, no redness or swelling.

Apical pulse is 64 and regular; lungs are clear. Abdomen is soft with BS present in all four quadrants. MAE. Pedal and radial pulses 2+. No edema. Skin is dry and warm. No bruises, abrasions, or cuts. He is able to stand and walk in his room with a normal gait. Braden score 23. J.R. has no drug allergies.

J.R. states that he lives alone in an apartment but has a girlfriend who visits frequently. His family lives about a half hour from him. He graduated from college 1 year ago with a degree in accounting and has a job working for a small accounting firm. He has felt a lot of stress lately because of work and has been working late many days. He gets 5 to 6 hours of sleep at night and often "eats on the run." Nothing else in his life has changed recently. He has not felt ill or had any other new symptoms. He first had seizures when he was a toddler. He has been on a variety of medications over the years. He sees his neurologist every 6 months and last had blood work 4 months ago. For the past 4 years, he has been taking carbamazepine 400 mg orally twice daily. His last seizure was 6 years ago, at which time phenobarbital was added, but it made him tired. When he was 2 years' seizure-free, the doctor took him off of it. He states he is worried about his job and what his co-workers saw today. He is also concerned about driving because he has to get himself to work. His girlfriend knows about his seizures but has never witnessed one because they met 2 years ago. She is coming to the hospital after work today.

8. From what J.R. has told you, what might have put him at a higher risk for a breakthrough seizure?

9. What three nursing diagnoses or patient problems might be included in your plan of care for J.R.?

10. With which members of the interprofessional team might you collaborate to address J.R.'s concerns about work and driving? Describe how each member of the team can contribute to J.R.'s care.

11. While you are taking VS at 1800, J.R. tells you he feels "funny" and begins to have another seizure. His girlfriend is at bedside. What important care should you provide?

ASSESSMENT UPDATE

The next morning, you are again assigned to care for J.R. You learn in report that he had a quiet night without further seizures and that he slept most of the evening and night. He expressed concern to the night nurse about how upset his girlfriend was yesterday after his seizure in the hospital. He states that "it was very scary for her, and she was crying."

Lab results (may vary by facility): *BMP: sodium 134 mEq/L; potassium 3.8; chloride 100 mEq/L; bicarbonate 22 mEq/L; BUN 22 mg/dL; creatinine 1.2 mg/dL; glucose 100 mg/dL*

CBC: *hemoglobin 15 g/dL; hematocrit 45%; white blood cells 8000 mm³; platelets 300,000 mm³*

Carbamazepine blood level 12 mcg/mL

LFT AST 35 units/L, ALT 38 units/L, AP 120 units/L, bilirubin 1.4 mg/dL

Lipid panel Total Cholesterol 220 mg/dL, HDL 70 mg/dL, LDL 150 mg/dL, Triglycerides 170 mg/dL

Urinalysis: *normal except positive for glucose, protein 12 mg/dL. EEG results are pending.*

New orders: *Discontinue previous carbamazepine orders.*

Carbamazepine 200 mg PO in the morning and 400 mg PO in the evening

Divalproex sodium 200 mg PO qid

12. Add J.R.'s patient data to the CCM in this book for Case Study 12 or in the CCM Creator on Evolve. For his medications, add the classification of each and why the patient is taking it. Include all lab values. Mark any abnormal value with and high ↑ or low ↓ arrow. Note the normal range for any abnormal lab values. Explain how each abnormal value relates to J.R.'s current medical condition.

13. What are your priority interventions as you care for J.R. today?

14. What will you tell J.R. about divalproex sodium and the reduction in dose of carbamazepine?

ASSESSMENT UPDATE

J.R. is being discharged on carbamazepine and divalproex. The social worker is working with J.R. on transportation for work. J.R. has spoken to his boss, discussed his illness, and will return to work next week. His girlfriend is coming to pick him and continues to be supportive of him. He has asked her to come to his next neurology appointment with him so that she can continue to learn about epilepsy.

15. What discharge instructions will you give J.R.?

16. Complete the CCM for Case Study 12 in this book or in the CCM Creator on Evolve for J.R. with an individualized plan of care for the three identified nursing diagnoses/patient problems based on J.R.'s assessment findings.

Medications

Carbamazepine 200 mg PO in the morning, 400 mg PO in the evening

Divalproex sodium 200 mg PO qid

IV Sites/Fluids/Rate

Saline lock 20 g in left forearm
Flush with 10 mL NS q 8 hr

Past Medical/Surgical History

Epilepsy since he was a toddler

Variety of anticonvulsants over the years

For the past 4 years, he has been taking only carbamazepine 400 mg bid.

Last seizure was 6 years ago, at which time phenobarbital was added, which made him tired.

At 2 years, seizure-free, the doctor took him off phenobarbitol.

Sees his neurologist every 6 months and last had blood work 4 months ago.

Conceptual Care Map

Student Name_____

Patient Initials ___J.R.___ Room # _____ Admission Date _____

CODE Status ___Full___ Today's Date _____

Age _24_ Gender _M_ Weight _82.7 kg (182lb)_ Height _177.8 cm (70 in)_

Braden Score _23_ Diet ___Adult regular___

Activity ___Up ad lib___ Religion _Roman Catholic_ Allergies _NKDA___

Admitting Diagnoses/Chief Complaint

Generalized tonic-clonic seizure

Assessment Data

Admitted to medical unit from ED. A co-worker called 911 after J.R. "fell to the floor and began shaking." When EMT arrived, the seizure had stopped. Another seizure started about 2 minutes later, so the decision was made to transport him to the ED.

Initial exam on medical unit at 1400, 3 hours after the seizures occurred: VS: T 36.2.5° C (97.2° F), BP 122/76, P 62 and regular, R 16 and unlabored. O$_2$ saturation 94% on RA. States his arms and legs hurt a bit; rates the pain at 2/10. A&Ox4. PERRLA. Head and neck exam are normal with no JVD. Says he still feels a bit "weird" from the seizures and correctly states the date but is unsure about the time. J.R. is answering questions appropriately and says he remembers "feeling funny" before the seizure but doesn't remember anything else until he was in the ambulance. Saline lock in left forearm, no redness or swelling.

Apical pulse 64 and regular; lungs are clear. Abdomen is soft with BS present in all four quadrants. MAE. Pedal and radial pulses 2+. No edema. Skin is dry and warm. No bruises, abrasions, or cuts. He is able to stand and walk in his room with a normal gait.

Lives alone in an apartment, has a girlfriend who visits frequently. Family lives about a half hour from him. Graduated from college 1 year ago with a degree in accounting and has a job working for a small accounting firm. Has felt a lot of stress lately because of work, and has been working late many days. Gets 5-6 hours of sleep at night and often "eats on the run." Nothing else has changed recently. Has not felt ill or had any other new symptoms. He states he is worried about his job and what his co-workers saw today. Also concerned about driving because he has to get himself to work. His girlfriend knows about his seizures but has never witnessed one because they met 2 years ago. She is coming to visit after work today.

Next morning: slept most of the evening and night. He expressed concern to the night nurse about how upset his girlfriend was yesterday after his seizure in the hospital. He states that "it was very scary for her, and she was crying."

Lab Values/Diagnostic Test Results

BMP

CBC

Misc Lab Values/Diagnostic Test Results

EEG pending

Carbamazepine blood level:

LFT:

Lipid panel:

Urinalysis:

Treatments

Seizure precautions

VS q 4 hr

Adult regular diet

I&O

Up ad lib

Labs pending: carbamazepine blood level, CBC, BMP, LFT, fasting lipid panel, and urinalysis

---

Primary Nursing Diagnosis	Nursing Diagnosis 2	Nursing Diagnosis 3
Supporting Data	Supporting Data	Supporting Data
STG/NOC	STG/NOC	STG/NOC
Interventions/NIC with Rationale	Interventions/NIC with Rationale	Interventions/NIC with Rationale
Rationale Citation/EBP	Rationale Citation/EBP	Rationale Citation/EBP
Evaluation	Evaluation	Evaluation

ⓔ An interactive version of the Conceptual Care Map is on Evolve.

CASE STUDY 13

Manuel Rodriguez

Name/s _____ Date _____

Patient Assignment

M.R. is a 43-year-old Hispanic male who has a follow-up appointment at the diabetic clinic. One and a half years ago, he was diagnosed with type 2 diabetes mellitus (DM). He has been to the emergency department (ED) twice in the past year for hyperglycemic episodes. M.R. is divorced and lives alone. He has a 16-year-old son who he sees frequently. His family history includes type 2 DM in both his father and paternal grandfather. M.R. was raised Roman Catholic but currently does not attend church. He has no allergies.

1300 VS: T 36.5° C (97.7° F), BP 138/88, P 76 and regular, R 20 and unlabored. O_2 saturation 96% on RA. Height 170.2 cm (67 in). Weight 95.5 kg (210 lb). BMI 32.9. Denies pain. A&O×4. PERRLA. Head & neck exam are normal with no JVD. Apical pulse is 76 and regular; lungs are clear. Abdomen is soft and round with BS present in all four quadrants. MAE. Peripheral pulses 2+. No edema. Skin is dry and warm. Normal gait.

Lab results: HbA_{1C} 10% (Lab results may vary by facility.)
Fingerstick blood glucose 200 mg/dL
Medications: metformin 850 mg PO bid.

1. What known risk factors did M.R. have for developing type 2 DM?

2. What data in M.R.'s assessment are of concern to you as the diabetic clinic nurse?

3. What is HbA_{1C}?

4. As the clinic nurse responsible for diabetic teaching, what questions will you ask M.R. to determine his symptoms and level of understanding of DM?

ASSESSMENT UPDATE

M.R. states that he is monitoring his blood glucose "a couple of times a day." He eats coffee and a muffin or bagel from the coffee shop for breakfast. Lunch is usually a sandwich and some chips delivered to his office, or a quick stop at a fast food restaurant. Dinner is something simple and quick if he is home, or pizza if he is out. He admits to snacking frequently on "things that probably aren't good for me because I feel hungry all the time." He states he does urinate frequently but thinks it is probably because he drinks large quantities of water and diet pop.

M.R. has been very busy at work and when he gets home, he often goes to the ball field to watch his son play baseball. He states that he is too exhausted after working and attending to family stuff to exercise. M.R. has taken his medication twice most days. He thinks he has missed two or three doses in the past month but is not sure if the missed doses are related to any symptoms. He does not have any wounds that he knows of but has had some tingling in his feet. His vision is a bit blurry sometimes at work. He notices it especially in the afternoon when he is tired. He states that it is hard to follow all these instructions with no one to help him.

At this clinic visit, glipizide 5 mg PO daily is added to his diabetic treatment regimen. Referrals are made to DM support group, counseling, dietitian and ophthalmologist.

5. What nursing diagnoses or patient problems might be included in your plan of care for M.R.?

6. What can the health care team do to help M.R. deal with DM and follow a healthy treatment plan?

7. What are the major diabetic teaching points that you would like to get across to M.R. during this visit? Use terminology that the patient will understand and include teaching about DM, dietary considerations, exercise, medications, blood glucose monitoring, symptoms of hypoglycemia and hyperglycemia, and complications of DM.

8. Outline the steps performed when performing a fingerstick blood glucose test.

9. What is the rationale behind sending M.R. for an ophthalmology consult?

10. Add M.R.'s patient data to the CCM in this book for Case Study 13 or in the CCM Creator on Evolve. In the CCM, prioritize three of the nursing diagnoses or problems from question 5 and formulate an individualized plan of care for M.R. during this clinic visit. Include diagnostic statements; supporting data; measurable, patient-centered goals; and interventions with EBP rationales. Evaluate the plan of care using the assessment update below at the appointment 1 week later.

One week later: M.R. has his weekly follow-up appointment at the diabetic clinic. 1430 VS: T 36.8° C (98.2° F), BP 134/84, P 72 and regular, R 20 and unlabored. O$_2$ saturation 98% on RA. Weight 95 kg (209 lb). BMI 32.7. There are no changes in his physical exam from 1 week ago. He states that he has started walking 10 minutes every morning and 10 minutes every evening.

He met with the dietitian. They discussed his usual diet and then made a list of healthy choices within his cultural and social parameters. The discussion included a list of choices for breakfast, lunch, and dinner, some of which he can buy already prepared fresh or frozen at the grocery store. He feels overwhelmed by having to change "so much all at once." He says he is "not much of a cook or shopper." He hasn't been to the grocery store since the appointment but will get there soon. He has been trying to snack less, eating fruits and carrots when he does snack, and is choosing different items when he eats out that better fit the plan he and the dietitian discussed.

He has been checking his blood glucose level around three times a day and it is usually between 140 to 180 mg/dL. He states that he filled the new prescription immediately and has been diligent about taking his medications. He expresses concern over being able to handle all of this and hopes that the support group meetings will help. The group meets every other week and the next meeting is this week.

11. What positive changes has M.R. made during the past week?

12. What are your priorities as you encourage M.R. and prepare diabetic teaching for today?

One month later: M.R. has his weekly follow-up appointment at the diabetic clinic. M.R. brought his 16-year-old son with him to the appointment because his son is interested in learning more about DM. 1530 VS: T 36.5° C (97.7° F), BP 130/78, P 68 and regular, R 16 and unlabored. Weight 91.8 kg (202 lb). BMI 31.6. His physical exam is unchanged. He says he has not had any episodes of tingling in his toes or blurred vision lately. He is testing his blood glucose levels four times a day and they are running between 130 to 150 mg/dL. He has continued walking and is excited to have lost 3.6 kg (8 lb) in the past month. He feels that he still has some changes to make in his eating habits but is doing better than before. He states that it finally sank in last month that this was serious and he does not want to get sicker. He thinks a lot about his grandfather who died when M.R. was a teenager. As far back as he can remember his grandfather was an amputee because of DM. He is trying to follow the instructions to set an example for his son but states "it is really hard to follow it all." He has been to two support group meetings and was interested in some of the suggestions that other patients found helpful.

13. Evaluate M.R.'s plan of care based on this week's assessment.

14. In the table below, reevaluate his plan of care based on three short-term goals (STG) set in the CCM with the data from this visit.

STG Patient will test blood glucose levels 4 times daily within the next week.	STG Patient will lose 2.3 kg (5 lb) per month until BMI is <25.0.	STG Patient will report healthy snacking at next clinic visit. Modified to a long-term goal of HbA_{1c} <7%.
EVALUATION	EVALUATION	EVALUATION

15. What positive reinforcement can you give to M.R. about the past month?

16. In what areas will you support M.R. to continue to work?

17. What teaching is appropriate for M.R.'s son?

Medications

Metformin 850 mg PO bid
Glipizide 5 mg PO daily

IV Sites/Fluids/Rate

Past Medical/Surgical History

Family history of type 2 DM: father and
 paternal grandfather
Type 2 DM for 1½ years
ED twice in past year for hyperglycemic
 episodes.

Conceptual Care Map

Student Name_____

Patient Initials __M.R.__ Room # _____ Admission Date __outpatient__

CODE Status _____ Today's Date _____

Age _43_ Gender _M_ Weight _95.5 kg (210 lb)_ Height _170.2 cm (67 in)_

Braden Score ____ Diet _____

Activity _____ Religion _Roman Catholic__ Allergies _none___

Admitting Diagnoses/Chief Complaint

Type 2 Diabetes mellitus /Follow-up appointment at diabetes clinic

Assessment Data

VS: T 36.5° C (97.7° F), BP 138/88, P 76 and regular, R 20 and
 unlabored. O_2 saturation 96% on RA. BMI 32.9. Denies pain. A&Ox4.
 PERRLA. Head & neck exam are normal with no JVD. Apical pulse is
 76 and regular; lungs are clear. Abdomen is soft and round with BS
 present in all four quadrants. MAE. Peripheral pulses 2+. No edema.
 Skin is dry and warm. Normal gait. M.R. is divorced, lives alone, 16-
 year-old son who he sees frequently.

M.R. states that he is monitoring his blood glucose "a couple of times a
 day." Eats: coffee and a muffin or bagel from for breakfast; a
 sandwich and some chips, or a quick stop at a fast food restaurant for
 lunch; something simple and quick, or pizza for dinner. Snacks
 frequently on "things that probably aren't good for me because I feel
 hungry all the time." Urinates frequently and drinks large quantities of
 water and diet pop.

Very busy at work and when he gets home, he often goes to the ball
 field to watch his son play baseball. He states that he is too
 exhausted after working and attending to family stuff to exercise.
 Takes his medication twice most days, missed two or three doses in
 the past month. No wounds but has had some tingling in his feet. His
 vision is a bit blurry sometimes at work, especially in the afternoon
 when he is tired. He states that it is hard to follow all these
 instructions with no one to help him.

Lab Values/Diagnostic Test Results

BMP

CBC

Misc Lab Values/Diagnostic Test Results

HbA_{1C} 10%
Fingerstick blood glucose 200 mg/dL

Treatments

Diabetic teaching

Primary Nursing Diagnosis	Nursing Diagnosis 2	Nursing Diagnosis 3
Supporting Data	Supporting Data	Supporting Data
STG/NOC	STG/NOC	STG/NOC
Interventions/NIC with Rationale	Interventions/NIC with Rationale	Interventions/NIC with Rationale
Rationale Citation/EBP	Rationale Citation/EBP	Rationale Citation/EBP
Evaluation	Evaluation	Evaluation

ⓔ An interactive version of the Conceptual Care Map is on Evolve.

CASE STUDY 14

Jack Weingart

Name/s _____ Date _____

Patient Assignment

J.W. is 1-day postoperative robot-assisted prostatectomy for prostate cancer. He is married, 78 years old, and plays golf one to two times per week throughout the year. J.W. is a full code with allergies to fire ants and bees with an activity order of up ad lib. His diet is adult general. He is 188 cm (74 in) tall and weighs 95.4 kg (210 lb). J.W.'s religious preference is Jewish.

Initial Assessment

0730 VS: T 37.8° C (100° F), BP 152/74, P 68 and regular, R 16 and unlabored with a pain level of 2 to 3 in the groin area and at the tip of the penis where his urinary catheter is inserted. J.W. describes the pain as dull and nonradiating that goes away when he does not move around. His O_2 saturation is 98% on RA. J.W. is A&O×4, PERRLA, with a Braden score of 21. Lungs are clear bilaterally. Abdomen is soft and slightly tender with BS×4. J.W. has a triple-lumen urinary catheter in place for continuous bladder irrigation. He has a midline incision over his left knee from a total knee replacement 5 years ago. Pedal pulses are 2+ bilaterally. J.W. has a 20-gauge saline lock in his left hand. He does not require help with ADL, but has been instructed to seek assistance for getting out of bed and ambulating.

1. Name three postoperative interventions that should be implemented to prevent J.W. from developing pneumonia. Provide a rationale for each and add each to the treatment subsection of the CCM for Case Study 14 in this book or in the CCM Creator on Evolve.

2. List four postoperative interventions to prevent deep vein thrombosis (DVT) or venous thromboembolism (VTE) formation. Add each of them to the treatment or medication subsection of J.W.'s plan of care on the CCM.

3. The UAP assigned to help care for J.W. reports that the urine in the collection bag is quite red and contains some deeper red floating debris. Choose the best initial response from the options below, and then write a detailed explanation that you would give to the UAP.
   a. "Thank you for telling me. I will call his PCP when I am done passing meds."
   b. "Okay. Please collect some of the urine from the bag for urinalysis."
   c. "I appreciate your letting me know. Does it appear bloodier than earlier?"
   d. "Alright. I will check to see if his hemoglobin and hematocrit are elevated."

4. Explain the step-by-step procedure for initiating and performing continuous bladder irrigation.

5. What interventions related to closed bladder irrigation can UAP perform?

6. What lab results would be important for you as the RN to monitor related to J.W.'s bleeding postoperatively? Provide a rationale for your answer.

7. On what type of precautions should J.W. be placed? Give a minimum of two reasons for implementing each precaution with J.W.

8. Identify the appropriate nursing diagnosis or patient problem statement related to the precautions on which J.W. should be placed, and add it your CCM for J.W. Develop the corresponding areas of J.W.'s plan of care relative to the nursing diagnosis or patient problem statement you wrote.

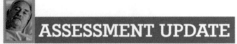

ASSESSMENT UPDATE

On his second postoperative day, J.W.'s assessment findings include: VS: T 37° C (98.6° F), BP 145/70, P 64 and regular, R 18 and unlabored with a report of mild groin pain, severity of 1-2/10. J.W. is ordered acetaminophen 650 mg PO q 4 hr PRN, which he is requesting 2 to 3 times per day while awake. His latest CBC results are: WBC 7000 mm³, Hgb 12 g/dL, Hct 40%, PLT 250 x 10⁹/L. His urine is becoming more pink than red. He walked to the bathroom to complete his ADL in the morning and ambulated about 50 feet on the nursing unit with assistance in the early afternoon.

9. Add the acetaminophen order to J.W.'s CCM. Include the classification of the medication and the reason he is receiving it.

10. What is the maximum daily dosage of acetaminophen?

11. What is the major reason why people should not take more than the recommended daily dose of acetaminophen?

12. Document J.W.'s CBC results in the CCM. Interpret the abnormal results by using arrows to indicate when findings are out of normal range, and provide the normal range and an explanation for each abnormality.

13. While J.W.'s catheter is in place, the PCP requests a urinalysis. Briefly explain the procedure for obtaining a urine sample from an indwelling catheter.

14. Can the collection of urine from a urinary catheter port be delegated to UAP?

15. J.W. and his wife are concerned about his diagnosis of prostate cancer and its effect on his typical daily activities and their ability for intimacy. What discussion topics and/or referrals would be most helpful to provide support surrounding their concerns?

16. Identify a second nursing diagnosis or patient problem statement for J.W. based on the concerns of him and his wife. Develop a plan of care in J.W.'s CCM to address the nursing diagnosis or patient problem.

Medications

IV Sites/Fluids/Rate
20-gauge saline lock LH

Past Medical/Surgical History
S/P robot-assisted prostatectomy
Left total knee replacement 5 years ago

Conceptual Care Map
Student Name_____
Patient Initials __J.W.__ Room # _____ Admission Date _____
CODE Status __Full___ Today's Date _____
Age _78_ Gender _M_ Weight _95.4 kg (210 lb)_ Height __188 cm (74 in)__
Braden Score _21_ Diet __Adult General___ Activity _Up Ad Lib____
Religion _____Jewish_____ Allergies __Fire ants, bees____

Admitting Diagnoses/Chief Complaint
Prostate Cancer

Assessment Data
0730 VS: T 37.8° C (100° F), BP 152/74, P 68 and regular, R 16 and
 unlabored; pain level of 2 to 3 in the groin area and at the tip of the
 penis where his urinary catheter is inserted. Describes the pain as
 dull and nonradiating that goes away when he doesn't move around.
 O$_2$ saturation 98% on RA.

A&Ox4, PERRLA. Lungs clear bilaterally. Abdomen soft and slightly
 tender with BSx4.

Triple-lumen urinary catheter in place for continuous bladder irrigation.
 Midline incision over his left knee. Pedal pulses are 2+ bilaterally.

Does not require help with ADLs; instructed to seek assistance for
 getting out of bed and ambulating

Married, plays golf one to two times per week

Lab Values/Diagnostic Test Results
BMP

CBC

Misc Lab Values/Diagnostic Test Results

Treatments

Primary Nursing Diagnosis	Nursing Diagnosis 2	Nursing Diagnosis 3
Supporting Data	**Supporting Data**	**Supporting Data**
STG/NOC	**STG/NOC**	**STG/NOC**
Interventions/NIC with Rationale	**Interventions/NIC with Rationale**	**Interventions/NIC with Rationale**
Rationale Citation/EBP	**Rationale Citation/EBP**	**Rationale Citation/EBP**
Evaluation	**Evaluation**	**Evaluation**

ⓔ An interactive version of the Conceptual Care Map is on Evolve.

CASE STUDY

15
Nicole Kaiser

Name/s _____ Date _____

Patient Assignment

N.K. is a 21-year-old female who was brought to the emergency department (ED) by the emergency medical technician (EMT) squad at 1100. She is a college junior who fainted and fell when she stood up at the end of a class. The professor called 911. The EMT squad reports to the ED nurse that when they arrived, N.K. was pale but awake and talking. Her pulse was 124, and she had a 2-inch laceration on her lower right arm. Another student reported to the squad that N.K. hit her arm on the desk when she fell and that her books went flying out of her arms.

1. As the ED nurse, what questions will you ask N.K.?

2. What initial assessments will be important?

Initial Assessment

N.K. states that she felt dizzy a couple of days ago, but she sat down and did not faint. Nothing hurts besides her right arm, and she does not think she bumped anything else. N.K. says that she is usually healthy but admits to being very tired lately and can barely make it up steps without "breathing hard." She is not sure if her pulse has been fast because she "doesn't know how to take it," but she can sometimes feel thumping in her chest. She has not had any bleeding except during her period, which she says has been "really heavy lately." N.K. says that she eats in her apartment most of the time and that since she moved out of the dorm, she does not eat full meals very often.

VS: T 36.5° C (97.7° F), BP 90/58, P 120 and regular, R 24 and labored with exertion. O_2 saturation 95% on RA. Denies pain, except in lower right arm near the laceration, which she says stings. She rates the pain at a 3/10. Height 167.6 cm (66 in). Weight 50.9 kg (112 lb). N.K. is A&O×4, PERRLA. Lungs clear. Apical pulse is 122 and regular. Abdomen is soft and nontender. BS active in four quadrants. Skin pale, warm, and dry. Active range of motion (ROM) in all four extremities is normal. Two-inch laceration on right lower arm covered with gauze by the EMT. The wound is still oozing a small amount of bright red blood. Pedal pulses 2+ bilaterally. NKDA.

3. What is N.K.'s BMI?

4. Which assessment findings are of concern?

5. What safety precautions are put into place during N.K.'s stay in the ED?

 ASSESSMENT UPDATE

1200: The ED physician examined N.K., cleansed her wound, applied skin adhesive to the wound, and ordered an EKG and lab work: CBC, BMP, serum iron, ferritin, prealbumin. She is being held in the ED pending the test results. She states that she is "willing to do whatever it takes to feel better because it was scary to pass out." She has cried on and off since arriving in the emergency room and is anxious about the test results, stating she hopes they "don't find anything serious wrong."

N.K. is resting in an ED room. Her roommate is at bedside. Blood has been drawn for the ordered lab tests. EKG shows normal sinus rhythm with tachycardia.

Lab results: BMP normal; CBC: WBC 6000/mm³, Hgb 8 g/dL, Hct 30%, Platelets 300,000 × 10⁹/L. Fe 48 mcg/dL, ferritin 8 ng/mL, prealbumin 25 mg/dL. (Lab results may vary by facility.)

6. How would you explain the EKG results to N.K.?

7. From N.K.'s assessment data, what is the probable cause of her abnormal lab values?

8. Interpret the lab results and place the interpretation on the CCM for Case Study 15 in this book or in the CCM Creator on Evolve for N.K.

9. List at least 3 nursing diagnoses or patient problems that are appropriate for N.K.

10. Prioritize the nursing diagnoses and complete the Conceptual Care Map (CCM) for N.K. Complete the first page data collection section. Prioritize three of the nursing diagnoses you listed in the previous question and formulate an individualized plan of care for N.K. Evaluate the plan of care when N.K. is discharged from the ED.

11. Your shift is ending and you need to prepare a handoff report to the evening shift nurse. Write a handoff report in SBAR format.

ASSESSMENT UPDATE

The ED physician has diagnosed N.K. with iron-deficiency anemia, based on her history and her lab work. The physician is going to discharge N.K. later this evening. She will be referred to her gynecologist for an ultrasound and further testing to investigate the heavy periods. A dietitian has been consulted and will meet with N.K. before she leaves the hospital.

12. What type of diet will the dietitian most likely recommend for N.K.'s iron-deficiency anemia?

13. What other recommendations might the dietitian have for N.K., given her BMI?

ASSESSMENT UPDATE

1700: N.K.'s discharge orders include: Ferrous sulfate 300 mg PO daily. Diet: high iron diet. Follow-up with gynecologist as soon as possible for heavy menstrual periods. Follow-up with PCP in 2 weeks for iron-deficiency anemia. Wound care protocol for skin adhesive closure.

14. What teaching will you provide to N.K. when you discharge her? Include teaching about iron-deficiency anemia, the new medication, wound care, and dietary recommendation.

15. N.K. states that she understands the diet instructions, but does not cook much and is concerned about having time to prepare meals that are healthy. What suggestions can you give her about food choices and preparation?

16. What follow-up care can N.K. expect from her gynecologist and PCP? How will they monitor her treatment?

Medications

IV Sites/Fluids/Rate

Past Medical/Surgical History

Dizzy a couple of days ago
Heavy menstrual periods

Conceptual Care Map

Student Name_____

Patient Initials __N.K.__ Room # __3__ Admission Date _____

CODE Status _____ Today's Date _____

Age _21_ Gender _F_ Weight _50.9 kg (112 lb)_ Height _167.6 cm (66 in)___

Braden Score _____ Diet _____ Activity _Up with assistance_

Religion _____ Allergies__NKDA_____

Admitting Diagnoses/Chief Complaint

Fainted and fell/dizzy and laceration on arm

Assessment Data

1100: N.K. was brought to the ED by the EMT squad. She is a college junior who fainted and fell when she stood up at the end of a class. The professor called 911. The EMT squad reports that when they arrived at the college, N.K. was pale but awake and talking. Pulse was 124. She had a 2-inch laceration on her lower right arm. Another student reported that N.K. hit her arm on the desk when she fell and that her books went flying out of her arms.

N.K. states that she felt dizzy a couple of days ago, but she sat down and did not faint. Nothing hurts besides her right arm, and she doesn't think she bumped anything else. N.K. says that she is usually healthy but admits to being very tired lately and can barely make it up steps without "breathing hard." She is not sure if her pulse has been fast because she "doesn't know how to take it," but she can sometimes feel thumping in her chest. She hasn't had any bleeding except during her period, which she says has been "really heavy lately." N.K. says that she eats in her apartment most of the time, and that since she moved out of the dorm, she doesn't eat full meals very often.

VS: T 36.5 C (97.7° F), BP 90/58, P 120 and regular, R 24 and labored with exertion. O$_2$ saturation 95% on RA. Denies pain, except in lower right arm near the laceration, which she says stings. She rates the pain at a 3/10. N.K. is A&Ox4, PERRLA. Lungs clear. Apical pulse is 122 and regular. Abdomen is soft and nontender. BS active in all four quadrants. Skin is pale, warm, and dry. Active ROM in all four extremities is normal. Two-inch laceration on right lower arm, covered with gauze by the EMT. The wound is still oozing a small amount of bright red blood. Pedal pulses 2+ bilaterally.

1200: The ED physician examined N.K., cleansed her wound, and applied skin adhesive to the wound. She is being held in the ED pending the test results. States that she is "willing to do whatever it takes to feel better because it was scary to pass out." She has cried on and off since arriving in the emergency room and is anxious about the test results, stating she hopes they "don't find anything serious wrong."

N.K. is resting in an ED room. Her roommate is at bedside. Blood has been drawn for the ordered lab tests.

Lab Values/Diagnostic Test Results

BMP: normal

CBC
6000/mm^3 8 g/dL   300,000 x 10^9/L
30%

Misc Lab Values/Diagnostic Test Results

Fe 48 mcg/dL
Ferritin 8 ng/mL
Prealbumin 25 mg/dL
EKG: normal sinus rhythm with tachycardia

Treatments

Wound care
Fall precautions
Up with assistance
Call light within reach
CBC, BMP, serum iron, ferritin, prealbumin
Hold in ED pending lab results
Consult with dietitian

Primary Nursing Diagnosis	Nursing Diagnosis 2	Nursing Diagnosis 3
Supporting Data	Supporting Data	Supporting Data
STG/NOC	STG/NOC	STG/NOC
Interventions/NIC with Rationale	Interventions/NIC with Rationale	Interventions/NIC with Rationale
Rationale Citation/EBP	Rationale Citation/EBP	Rationale Citation/EBP
Evaluation	Evaluation	Evaluation

e An interactive version of the Conceptual Care Map is on Evolve.

CASE STUDY 16

Michael Mills

Name/s _____   **Date** _____

[handwritten: A&O = alert & oriented — (x1)–(x4) – alert oriented to place time and person. oriented self or person]

Patient Assignment

M.M. is a 25-year-old African American admitted to the hospital yesterday for sickle cell crisis (SCC). This is the second time he has been hospitalized in the past 6 months. He is a full code with allergies to aspirin and sulfa drugs. His diet is adult general, and he has a Braden score of 19. He is allowed up ad lib. M.M. is 180 cm (71 in) tall and weighs 60.4 kg (133 lb). His religion preference is Baptist. Recently he was hired at his dream job as a mechanical engineer, and is extremely concerned about missing work.

Initial Assessment

[handwritten margin notes: 120/80; 60–100 beats min; 12–20 beat min; abnormal breathing; absent or decrease in sound (if air flow to part of the lung); ↓ or absent of bowel sound; Normal 60–100]

0715 VS T 38.4° C (101.1° F), BP 107/64, P 70 and regular, R 18 and unlabored. O_2 saturation 94% on 2 L O_2 per NC. Pain of 9/10, described as diffuse throughout his body. A&O×4, lungs are clear in the upper lobes and diminished in the lower lobes bilaterally. No cough. Apical 70 bpm. Abdomen is tender and firm with hypoactive BS×4. LBM 2 days ago. Complaint of general weakness and constipation. Urine is clear and yellow. MAE. Nonpitting edema of the feet and ankles with pedal pulses of 1+ bilaterally. He requests that the lights be left off in his room. M.M. stays in bed, except for ADL and using the bathroom because of his pain. He has a past history of cholecystectomy 3 years ago.

M.M. has a peripherally inserted central catheter (PICC) line in his upper left arm that is patent with a transparent dressing in place that is signed and dated. His PCA of hydromorphone 1 mg/mL 0.9% normal saline (NS), 0.2 mg q 10 min to 1.4 mg/hr does not seem to be controlling his pain. He has an 18-gauge intracath in his right forearm into which his programmed IV of $D_5\frac{1}{2}NS$ is infusing at 150 mL/hr. He is ordered to receive 1 unit of packed red blood cells (PRCs), Heparin 5000 units subcut q 8 hr, Acetaminophen 650 mg q 4 hr PO PRN, and bisacodyl 30 mg PO daily. His morning BMP and CBC results are pending. M.M.'s treatment orders include falls precautions, I&O, knee-high antiembolic stockings, and SCDs.

1. Sickle cell anemia is the most severe form of sickle cell disease (SCD). Briefly explain what causes sickle cell anemia.

2. Describe the difference between sickle cell traits (SCT) and SCD.

3. What cultures or populations are more prone to have SCT or SCD?

4. List a minimum of three precipitating factors that may lead to sickle cell crisis.

5. What are the clinical manifestations of sickle cell crisis? Highlight the ones that M.M. is exhibiting.

6. Explain how to assess for skin color abnormalities on a person with dark skin.

7. What are some questions that you should ask M.M. to determine the extent of his support system available to help him cope with sickle cell disease?

M.M.'s morning lab results are as follows:

BMP
Na⁺ 140 mEq/L — Na^+ 140 mEq/L
K⁺ 3.6 mEq/L — K^+ 3.6 mEq/L
Cl⁻ 105 mEq/L — Cl^- 105 mEq/L
CO_2 26 mEq/L
BUN 12 mg/dL
Creatinine 0.94 mg/dL
BS 109 mg/dL

CBC
WBC 18×10^9/L
Hgb 6.7 g/dL
Hct 20.1%
Plt 372×10^9/L

8. Begin M.M.'s care plan by entering all of his assessment, medication, IV, lab, and treatment data into the CCM for Case Study 16 in this book or in the CCM Creator on Evolve. Be sure to add required information for all medications and abnormal laboratory results.

9. M.M. is only 25 years old. List a minimum of three reasons for his being on falls precautions.

10. Provide a rationale for M.M. being on D₅½NS at 150 mL/hr.

11. M.M. is on 2 L of O_2 per NC. Briefly explain the pathophysiology in sickle cell crisis that may require individuals to have supplemental oxygen therapy.

12. M.M. is reporting a pain level of 9/10 despite being on hydromorphone PCA. What actions should you take to address his pain?

13. Sometimes patients in sickle cell crisis are labeled as "drug-seeking." What strategies should nurses implement to address the pain of patients in SCC and avoid a judgmental attitude?

14. Explain the step-by-step procedure for administering blood products.

15. After reviewing all of M.M.'s assessment data, identify a minimum of five nursing diagnoses or patient problems that are appropriate for M.M. right now, and provide a rationale for choosing each one.

16. Select two physical and one psychosocial nursing diagnoses or patient problems that you identified for M.M. at the present time, and complete your CCM plan of care for Case Study 16. Make sure to include all aspects of the nursing process in your work.

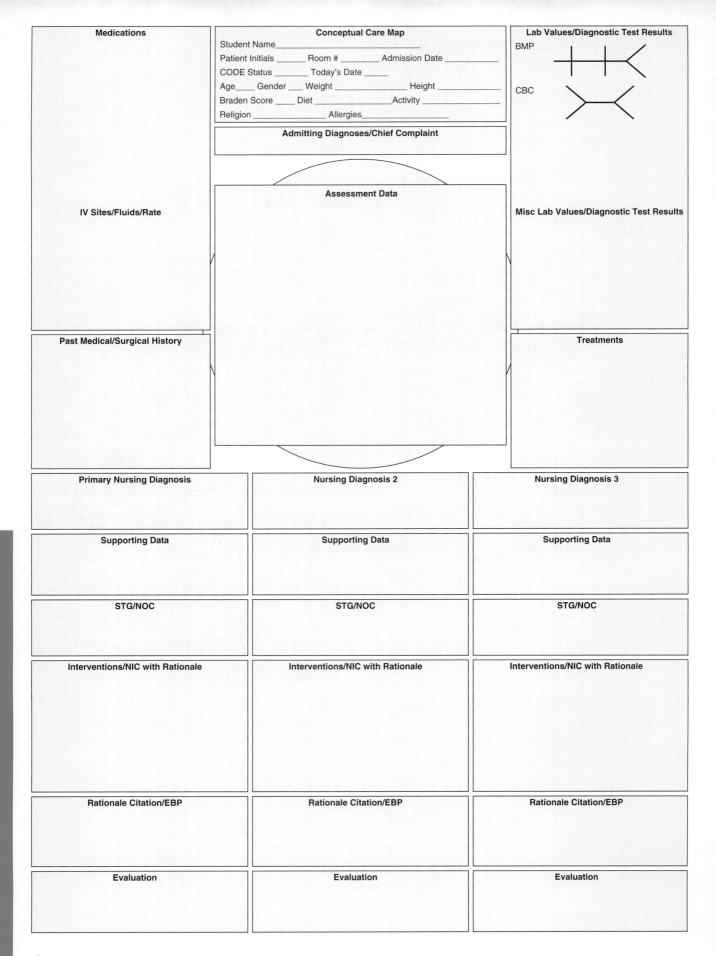

Conceptual Care Map

Medications

Lab Values/Diagnostic Test Results

BMP

CBC

Student Name_____

Patient Initials _____ Room # _____ Admission Date _____

CODE Status _____ Today's Date _____

Age_____ Gender ____ Weight _____ Height _____

Braden Score _____ Diet _____ Activity _____

Religion _____ Allergies_____

Admitting Diagnoses/Chief Complaint

Assessment Data

IV Sites/Fluids/Rate

Misc Lab Values/Diagnostic Test Results

Past Medical/Surgical History

Treatments

Primary Nursing Diagnosis	Nursing Diagnosis 2	Nursing Diagnosis 3
Supporting Data	Supporting Data	Supporting Data
STG/NOC	STG/NOC	STG/NOC
Interventions/NIC with Rationale	Interventions/NIC with Rationale	Interventions/NIC with Rationale
Rationale Citation/EBP	Rationale Citation/EBP	Rationale Citation/EBP
Evaluation	Evaluation	Evaluation

ⓔ An interactive version of the Conceptual Care Map is on Evolve.

CASE STUDY 17

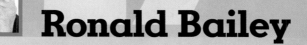

Ronald Bailey

Name/s _____ Date _____

Patient Assignment

R.B. is a 63-year-old male admitted to the nursing unit yesterday with acute exacerbation of chronic obstructive pulmonary disease (COPD). He has a history of HTN. He has NKDA, is a full code, and is on a low-salt diet. His Braden score is 22 and his activity is as tolerated. He is married with three grown children and four grandchildren. He works full time as a CPA in an accounting firm.

Initial Assessment

0700 VS T 38.9° C (102° F), BP 142/84, P 78 and regular, R 22 and labored. O_2 saturation 93% on 2 L O_2 per NC. Denies pain. A&O×4, DOE, wheezes and crackles are audible on auscultation, productive cough, and greenish sputum. Complaint of chest tightness. Apical pulse 80 bpm. Abdomen is soft and nontender with BS×4. Urine is clear and light yellow. MAE. Pedal pulses are 1+ bilaterally. Capillary refill >3 seconds. R.B. has a 20-gauge saline lock in his left hand. He becomes winded with any activity and requires short breaks while completing his activities of daily living (ADL). His medications include prednisolone 40 mg PO q AM, levofloxacin 750 mg IV daily, hydrochlorothiazide 12.5 mg PO daily, and captopril 25 mg PO bid. Orders include respiratory therapy 3×/day, falls precautions, O_2-2 L per NC to maintain >92% sat, CBC, BMP, and arterial blood gases (ABGs) daily and PRN, Accu-Check q 8 hr, saline lock, daily weights, I&O.

1. What two obstructive airway diseases are most often categorized as COPD? Which additional airway disease is sometimes encompassed within the broad category of COPD and may be a contributing factor in the development of COPD?

2. Identify the primary risk factor for COPD and a minimum of three additional risk factors.

3. Write a minimum of three interview questions that you should ask R.B. while collecting a health history.

4. Explain the etiologic difference between wheezes and crackles.

5. Barrel chest is one of the clinical manifestations of COPD. Explain what it is and what causes it to occur.

6. List additional signs and symptoms of COPD. Highlight or circle each one that R.B. is exhibiting.

7. Begin R.B.'s patient-centered plan of care by filling in the data organization and synthesis section of the CCM for Case Study 17 in this book or in the CCM Creator on Evolve. Be sure to include the classification and rationale for each ordered medication.

8. Provide a rationale for R.B. having blood glucose testing every 8 hours as he is not diabetic.

9. Two compensatory breathing techniques that patients with COPD use are sitting in a *tripod position* and *pursed-lip breathing*. Describe what the tripod position looks like and explain how it enhances breathing.

9a. Provide instructions for teaching pursed-lip breathing, and list a minimum of three reasons COPD patients would find pursed-lip breathing helpful.

10. What are the most common causes of acute exacerbation of COPD?

11. Identify at least four assessment findings and one medication order indicating that R.B.'s COPD exacerbation is the result of one of the most common causative factors?

ASSESSMENT UPDATE

While you are interviewing R.B. about his health history, he reports smoking one pack of cigarettes a day for 40 years and having tried to quit repeatedly without success. He states, "I would really like to break this habit. I know it is killing me!" His 0800 lab results, including ABGs after 10 minutes on RA are as follows:

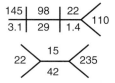

ABG
pH 7.24
PaCO$_2$ 56 mm Hg
HCO$_3$ 24 mEq/L
PaO$_2$ 58 mm Hg

12. Which BMP and CBC findings are abnormal? Provide a rationale for each abnormal result.

13. What are normal ABG levels for pH, $PaCO_2$, and HCO_3?

14. What do R.B.'s arterial blood gas results indicate? Provide a rationale for your answer and complete the lab values/diagnostic test results area of your CCM for R.B.

15. What two diagnostic tests would you expect to be ordered to evaluate the severity of R.B.'s current condition? Add them to the treatment section of your CCM for R.B.

ASSESSMENT UPDATE

Following scheduled respiratory therapy treatments, R.B.'s ABGs were repeated at 1900 with the following results after 10 minutes on RA:
ABG
pH 7.37
$PaCO_2$ 50 mm Hg
HCO_3 34 mEq/L
PaO_2 70 mm Hg

16. Provide a description of R.B.'s most recent ABG results and explain what has happened physiologically to achieve his current arterial blood gas levels.

17. What interventions would be helpful in response to R.B.'s request for help with smoking cessation? Identify a minimum of four.

18. Add all of R.B.'s lab results, their explanations, and updated assessment data to your CCM. Identify three nursing diagnoses for R.B. at this time and complete R.B.'s patient-centered plan of care.

Conceptual Care Map

Medications

IV Sites/Fluids/Rate

Past Medical/Surgical History

Student Name_____

Patient Initials _____ Room # _____ Admission Date _____

CODE Status _____ Today's Date _____

Age_____ Gender ____ Weight _____ Height _____

Braden Score _____ Diet _____ Activity _____

Religion _____ Allergies_____

Admitting Diagnoses/Chief Complaint

Acute exacerbation of COPD

Assessment Data

Lab Values/Diagnostic Test Results

BMP

CBC

Misc Lab Values/Diagnostic Test Results

Treatments

Primary Nursing Diagnosis	Nursing Diagnosis 2	Nursing Diagnosis 3
Supporting Data	Supporting Data	Supporting Data
STG/NOC	STG/NOC	STG/NOC
Interventions/NIC with Rationale	Interventions/NIC with Rationale	Interventions/NIC with Rationale
Rationale Citation/EBP	Rationale Citation/EBP	Rationale Citation/EBP
Evaluation	Evaluation	Evaluation

e An interactive version of the Conceptual Care Map is on Evolve.

CASE STUDY 18

William Ruby

Name/s _____ Date _____

Patient Assignment

W.R. is a 53-year-old executive who was diagnosed with atrial fibrillation 4 months ago. He had a successful cardioversion at that time. Three days ago, he began having "heart palpitations" and was admitted to the hospital an hour ago for R/O atrial fibrillation. He was placed on telemetry and falls precautions. He is a full code with an allergy to sulfa drugs and ragweed, and a Braden score of 23. W.R. is 180.3 cm (71 in) tall and weighs 69.5 kg (153 lb). He is ordered an adult general diet and allowed to be up ad lib.

Initial Assessment

1345 VS T 37° C (98.6° F), BP 128/74, P 124 and irregular, R 22 and unlabored. O_2 saturation 100% on RA. Denies pain. A&O×4. Lungs are clear on auscultation, no cough. Apical pulse 124 bpm. Abdomen is soft and nontender with BSx4. Urine is clear and light yellow. MAE. Dorsalis pedis pulses are 2+ bilaterally. Capillary refill <3 seconds. Complains of occasional dizziness and feeling faint when standing. States, "I began feeling really tired all the time a couple of days ago." W.R. has a 22-gauge saline lock in his right forearm (RFA).

W.R. is married with two children and one grandchild. He typically works between 60 and 70 hours a week as the CFO of an international company. His home medications include aspirin 325 mg PO and a multivitamin daily. Initial orders include telemetry, falls precautions, CBC and BMP daily, I&O. The on-call resident will be in to see W.R. within the hour and write medication orders.

1. Begin W.R.'s patient-centered care plan by completing the data organization and synthesis section of the CCM for Case Study 18 in this book or in the CCM Creator on Evolve.

2. Explain atrial fibrillation in terms that the patient and family would understand. Provide the links for two reputable websites that you could refer W.R. and his family to for additional information.

3. List a minimum of eight risk factors associated with atrial fibrillation.

4. Write three or more health history questions that you should ask W.R. while completing your assessment to help identify the etiology of his atrial fibrillation.

5. W.R. is on cardiac telemetry. Provide a brief explanation of telemetry that you would share with patients before placing them on it.

6. Identify the two most serious complications that can result from untreated atrial fibrillation and briefly explain their underlying etiologies.

7. Based on what you already know from W.R.'s assessment data, use your critical thinking skills to identify which electrocardiogram (ECG) strip is atrial fibrillation (AF) and which is normal sinus rhythm (NSR). Give a brief explanation of how someone who has not studied ECG analysis is able to tell the difference.

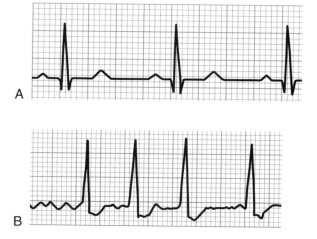

A

B

8. People may be asymptomatic with atrial fibrillation or they may experience a variety of signs and symptoms. List a minimum of four clinical manifestations that may be present with atrial fibrillation. Highlight those that W.R. is exhibiting.

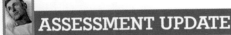

ASSESSMENT UPDATE

New orders for W.R. from the on-call resident include metoprolol ER 50 mg PO q AM, heparin IV 25,000 units in 250 mL of NS at 1200 units/hour, and warfarin 5 mg PO daily.

9. Update W.R.'s CCM to include his new medication orders.

10. What is the drug classification of heparin? What blood test is required to monitor the effect of heparin? What is the normal range for this blood test? What is considered the therapeutic range for patients on IV heparin? Briefly explain the reason for a difference between the normal and therapeutic range. Note the classification and reason for W.R. to take heparin in the medications area of your CCM. Add the associated lab test in the treatment area of your CCM.

11. At what rate should the infusion pump be set in order for W.R. to receive 1200 units of heparin per hour?

12. What is the drug classification of warfarin? What blood tests are required to monitor its effect? What would be the desired range for these blood test results while W.R. is receiving prophylactic warfarin treatment? What are the normal ranges? Note the classification and reason for W.R. to take warfarin in the medications area of your CCM. Add the associated lab tests in the treatment area of your CCM.

13. When a patient is placed on warfarin, what additional patient teaching is required?

14. What is the purpose of administering heparin IV and warfarin PO at the same time?

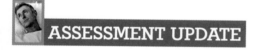

ASSESSMENT UPDATE

Thirty-six hours after initiation of his 12 units/hour IV heparin infusion, W.R.'s aPTT is 102 seconds.

15. As W.R.'s nurse, what three actions should you take immediately after receiving his aPTT results?

16. What is the classification of metoprolol? What will you monitor to determine if the metoprolol is effective?

17. List three potential life-threatening side effects and three common side effects of metoprolol.

18. What topics should be included in patient teaching for patients starting to take metoprolol?

19. Identify three nursing diagnoses for W.R. and complete your CCM to reflect his personalized plan of care.

Conceptual Care Map

Medications

IV Sites/Fluids/Rate

Past Medical/Surgical History

Conceptual Care Map

Student Name_____

Patient Initials _____ Room # _____ Admission Date _____

CODE Status _____ Today's Date _____ Age_____ Gender ___

Weight _____ Height _____

Braden Score _____ Diet _____Activity _____

Religion _____ Allergies_____

Admitting Diagnoses/Chief Complaint

Assessment Data

Lab Values/Diagnostic Test Results

BMP

CBC

Misc Lab Values/Diagnostic Test Results

Treatments

Primary Nursing Diagnosis	Nursing Diagnosis 2	Nursing Diagnosis 3
Supporting Data	Supporting Data	Supporting Data
STG/NOC	STG/NOC	STG/NOC
Interventions/NIC with Rationale	Interventions/NIC with Rationale	Interventions/NIC with Rationale
Rationale Citation/EBP	Rationale Citation/EBP	Rationale Citation/EBP
Evaluation	Evaluation	Evaluation

ⓔ An interactive version of the Conceptual Care Map is on Evolve.

CASE STUDY 19

Donald Bergman

Name/s_____ Date_____ _____

Patient Assignment

D.B. is a 67-year-old male who was admitted to the telemetry unit 1 day ago for medical management with a diagnosis of chronic heart failure (HF). D.B. has a 20-year history of hypertension and had an MI 6 years ago. He began having fatigue, tachycardia, and dependent bilateral lower extremity edema about 18 months ago, and was diagnosed with right ventricular HF. He was already taking enalapril for hypertension and was prescribed furosemide, potassium, and digoxin after his HF diagnosis. D.B.'s symptoms have worsened over the last month. Upon admission 1 day ago at 0800 VS: T 36.4° C (97.5° F), BP 156/98, P 126 and regular, R 36 and labored. O_2 saturation 88% on RA. He had 3+ pitting edema in his feet and ankles, dyspnea, tachycardia, JVD, and crackles bilaterally in his lungs. He stated that he has been unable to "get enough air," has been sleeping in the recliner, and has gained 5.5 kg (12 lb) in the past month. Admission weight 100 kg (220 lb), height 177.8 cm (70 in). He is a full code.

Admission Orders

Enalapril 5 mg PO bid, digoxin 0.25 mg PO daily, potassium 20 mEq PO daily, valsartan 40 mg PO bid, furosemide 0.1 mg/kg/hr continuous IV infusion, O_2 2L/min via nasal cannula to keep O_2 saturation at or above 92%. Bed rest with bathroom privileges. 2000-calorie DASH diet. 1500 mL/day fluid restriction. Daily weights. I&O. CBC, BMP, BNP, cardiac enzymes, ECG, echocardiogram, and chest x-ray. Admit to telemetry unit with 24-hour monitoring.

1. What signs and symptoms did D.B. have 18 months ago when he was diagnosed with right ventricular HF?

2. What are some other signs and symptoms of right HF?

3. What do his current signs and symptoms (3+ pitting edema in his feet and ankles, 5.5 kg (12 lb) weight gain, dyspnea, tachycardia, JVD, orthopnea, and crackles bilaterally in his lungs) indicate?

4. As you begin your shift, what are your assessment priorities?

5. List at least three assessment questions that you will ask D.B. during your first encounter.

6. The intravenous (IV) furosemide is sent from the pharmacy mixed in a 50 mL bag with a concentration of 50 mg furosemide in 50 mL of D_5W. What mL/hr will you set on the IV infusion pump for the furosemide 0.1 mg/kg/hr continuous IV infusion?

7. What dose of furosemide (mg/hr) is D.B. receiving?

ASSESSMENT UPDATE

During your morning assessment on day 2 at 0745: VS: T 37° C (98.6° F), BP 146/92, P 110 and regular, R 30 and labored. O_2 saturation 92% on 2L O_2 via nasal cannula. Denies pain but states he is just "uncomfortable and I still feel like I can't breathe." D.B. is A&Ox4, PERRLA. Bilateral crackles in all lung fields. Apical pulse is 110 and regular with a pulmonic murmur, no thrills. JVD present, no bruits heard on auscultation. Abdomen is soft, round, and nontender. BS present in all four quadrants. Skin warm and dry; skin on lower extremities taut and shiny. 2+ pitting edema of bilateral feet and ankles. Braden score 21. Pedal pulses 2+ bilaterally. MAE. IV infusing into 22-gauge catheter in right hand. No redness or swelling at site. Weight 98.2 kg (216 lb).

D.B. states that he is going to the bathroom "about every hour or two." He has the head of the bed almost flat with two pillows under his head. He is restless and anxious. He states that he has been too tired to do anything at home. D.B. tells you he has been married for 42 years. He says his wife will be visiting later. He has no known allergies. D.B. is Jewish, although he states he "hasn't felt well enough to go to Temple in a while."

8. Compared with D.B.'s admission assessment, which assessment findings are improved? To what do you attribute the improvement?

9. What will you do first for D.B. while you are in his room?

10. Outline the rationale for supplemental oxygen and the steps for administering oxygen through a nasal cannula.

11. D.B. asks why he has to be on "that special diet." Explain his diet to him.

12. D.B. is concerned about "how much I can have to drink." He states, "they gave me this piece of paper with numbers on it but I don't understand it." Explain the fluid restrictions to D.B. and formulate a plan for his restrictions so that he understands when he can have something to drink and how much.

1500-mL Fluid Restriction Plan for D.B.	
Fluid consumed at:	Amount in mL
Breakfast	
Lunch	
Dinner	
Between meals and medications	
Night shift	
IV fluids	

ASSESSMENT UPDATE

Today's lab and test results: CBC: normal
BMP: Sodium 136 mEq/L, Potassium 3.3 mEq/L; Chloride 97 mEq/L; Bicarb 24 mEq/L, BUN 18 mg/dL, Creatinine 1.2 mg/dL, Glucose 90 mg/dL
BNP 650 pg/dL
Cardiac enzymes: normal
ECG: sinus tachycardia 128 bpm
Echocardiogram: right and left ventricle hypertrophy, ejection fraction 38%, all valves functioning normally
Chest x-ray: cardiomegaly
(Lab results may vary by facility.)

13. Interpret D.B.'s abnormal lab results and enter them into the Conceptual Care Map (CCM) for Case Study 19 in this book or in the CCM Creator on Evolve.

ASSESSMENT UPDATE

1200: VS: T 36° C (96.8° F), BP 142/90, P 108 and regular, R 28 and labored. O₂ saturation 94% on 2L O₂ via nasal cannula. Denies pain. Physical assessment remains unchanged. Wife is at bedside and states she is "worried about him." D.B. says that his wife is supportive and she is the one who will be "cooking my meals." New order: Increase potassium to 20 mEq PO bid.

14. Write a priority nursing diagnosis statement or patient problem for D.B.

15. Write a patient-centered, measurable goal for the priority nursing diagnosis or patient problem.

16. Write at least two other nursing diagnoses statements or patient problems for D.B., then list several other potential nursing diagnoses.

17. What are some interventions that are important for D.B. today? Include medication administration and the six rights of medication administration.

18. Begin completing a CCM D.B. Complete the data section of the CCM. Use the priority nursing diagnostic statement or patient problem from question 14 along with the two other nursing diagnoses statements from question 16, and formulate an individualized plan of care for D.B. Include an evaluation of the short-term goals at this point in time.

19. When planning for D.B.'s discharge in a few days, his cardiologist is talking to him about cardiac rehabilitation. D.B. asks you to explain what the doctor means.

20. What other discharge teaching will be important for D.B. and his wife?

Conceptual Care Map

Medications

IV Sites/Fluids/Rate

Past Medical/Surgical History

Student Name_____
Patient Initials _____ Room # _____ Admission Date _____
CODE Status _____ Today's Date _____ Age_____ Gender ___
Weight _____ Height _____
Braden Score _____ Diet _____ Activity _____
_____ Religion _____ Allergies _____

Admitting Diagnoses/Chief Complaint

Assessment Data

Lab Values/Diagnostic Test Results

BMP

CBC

Misc Lab Values/Diagnostic Test Results

Treatments

Primary Nursing Diagnosis	Nursing Diagnosis 2	Nursing Diagnosis 3
Supporting Data	Supporting Data	Supporting Data
STG/NOC	STG/NOC	STG/NOC
Interventions/NIC with Rationale	Interventions/NIC with Rationale	Interventions/NIC with Rationale
Rationale Citation/EBP	Rationale Citation/EBP	Rationale Citation/EBP
Evaluation	Evaluation	Evaluation

ⓔ An interactive version of the Conceptual Care Map is on Evolve.

CASE STUDY 20

Catherine Abbott

Name/s_____ Date_____

Patient Assignment

C.A. is a 62-year-old female transferred to the cardiac step down unit from CCU. She was admitted 2 days ago to CCU following a myocardial infarction (MI). She saw her PCP in the office with symptoms of worsening fatigue and "indigestion." After an ECG her PCP sent her directly to the Emergency Department (ED). In the ED, her cardiac enzymes were elevated, indicative of a recent MI. She was transported to the cardiac intervention lab where a catheterization was performed. She had a 95% blockage in her left anterior descending coronary artery and a stent was inserted. C.A. has been slowly improving in CCU: ambulating short distances, on a cardiac diet, and alert but tired. VS have been stable. Braden score 22 and she has no known drug allergies.

History: Hypertension 15 years, treated with lisinopril
Hyperlipidemia 10 years, treated with atorvastatin
Cholecystectomy, age 50 years
Smoker 1 ppd × 25 years, quit 10 years ago
Menopause, age 48 years
Obesity: Height 157.5 cm (62 in), weight 100 kg (220 lb)

1. What is the difference in symptoms between men and women who are having a myocardial infarction?

2. What risk factors does C.A. have that would predispose her to an MI? What are some other risk factors that may contribute to development of MI? Which of these risk factors are modifiable through different lifestyle choices? Which are nonmodifiable?

3. What is C.A.'s BMI? What class of BMI is she?

4. What other information is important as you begin care for C.A.?

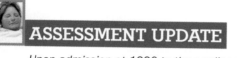

ASSESSMENT UPDATE

Upon admission at 1220 to the cardiac step down unit your assessment of C.A. includes: VS: T 37.4° C (99.3° F), BP 136/88, P 88 and regular, R 24 and slightly labored. O_2 saturation 96% on 2 L O_2 via nasal cannula. States that her leg still tingles a bit where the catheter was inserted, but she does not really have pain. States that she "doesn't feel that great." A&Ox4, but sleepy. PERRLA. Lungs clear. Apical pulse is 88 and regular. Abdomen is soft, round, and nontender. BS present in all four quadrants. Skin warm and dry. Small scab with a 10-cm ecchymotic area in right femoral area, no active bleeding. Pedal pulses 2+ bilaterally. 22-gauge saline lock in left hand. No redness or swelling at site. C.A.'s husband and adult daughter are in the room with her. They are conversing quietly. C.A. has advance directives on file and is a full code.

Current orders: Vital signs q 2 hr, up with assistance, SCDs while in bed, 24-hour telemetry monitoring, saline lock, flush with 10 mL NS q 8 hr. PT/INR in the morning. Medications: enoxaparin 120 mg subcut daily; warfarin 2 mg at 1600, call with INR for tomorrow's dosage; lisinopril 20 mg PO daily; atorvastatin 20 mg PO daily; morphine 2 mg IV push q 3 hr PRN for moderate to severe pain (4-10/10); acetaminophen 500 mg tablets, two tablets PO PRN for mild pain (1-3/10).

5. What is the rationale of administering enoxaparin and warfarin to C.A.?

6. What does "full code" mean? What other possible code status might a patient have?

7. What are advance directives?

1400: C.A.'s monitor begins to alarm and you enter her room. Her husband says, "She's complaining of not being able to breathe and her heart is pounding." According to the monitor, she is in ventricular tachycardia. You call a rapid response for her. As you begin to assess her, she goes into cardiac and respiratory arrest. After determining that she has no carotid pulse, you begin CPR just as the rapid response team is arriving. A code blue is called and the family is asked if they want to be in the room or wait outside of the room. The husband states, "I can't watch this." The daughter takes his arm and leads him out of the room.

The team works on C.A. for 20 minutes. She is intubated and bagged, defibrillated, chest compressions are performed, and medications are administered. The team is unable to restore her heartbeat. She is pronounced dead at 1425 by the resident physician on the rapid response team.

8. What critical steps did you take when C.A. first began to show signs of decline?

9. Which ECG strip represents ventricular tachycardia (VT)? How can VT lead to death?

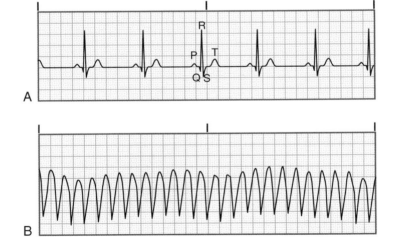

10. What signs need to be present to pronounce death?

ASSESSMENT UPDATE

The family has been waiting in the lounge. You and the physician enter the lounge and tell C.A.'s family that the team was unable to revive her and that she has died. The family is shocked and expresses disbelief. Because it is recorded on the chart that she is an organ donor, the physician approaches the family about organ donation. C.A.'s daughter states that "mom would want to help others." The husband begins crying and states, "I don't want anyone to take pieces of her. Just let her rest in peace." The two family members begin arguing about organ donation and the daughter leaves the room upset. The husband refuses to sign the forms for organ donation.

11. Who decides whether a patient can be an organ donor: the deceased patient who gave the hospital a copy of a signed organ donor card or the husband? What should your response be to the husband about organ donation and his refusal to sign the forms?

12. What are Kubler-Ross's stages of grief? How do you see them manifested by the family of C.A.?

13. What postmortem care should be performed?

ASSESSMENT UPDATE

The daughter returns and is crying. She hugs her dad and tells him she does not want to argue. Both family members express concern that C.A. died without having last rites. The husband asks if there is a priest that can come and give his wife last rites because they are Catholic. He states, "I don't know what could have happened. She was getting better." He asks the doctor how they can find out what happened and is told that an autopsy will be performed. The daughter asks if they can say goodbye to C.A. now.

14. What difference in postmortem care is necessary if the patient is having an autopsy?

15. The room has been straightened, C.A. has been bathed, and equipment from the rapid response team removed. You take the family in to see C.A. What therapeutic communication techniques will you use as the family sees their deceased loved one?

16. The priest enters the room while the family is saying goodbye and you are standing with the family. He begins praying with the family and performing last rites. You are not Catholic. What should you do next?

17. Because you are now caring for the patient's family, what nursing diagnoses or problems are appropriate as you support them? Prioritize a list of at least three problems or nursing diagnoses.

18. What interventions are appropriate for the family as you care for them after C.A.'s death?

19. Complete a CCM for Case Study 20 in this book or in the CCM Creator on Evolve for C.A.'s family. Enter all of the data for C.A. and her family from the case study. Formulate a plan of care for the family members after C.A.'s death.

20. What care is available for nurses and other staff members who are caring for dying patients or have experienced the sudden death of a patient?

Conceptual Care Map

Medications

IV Sites/Fluids/Rate

Past Medical/Surgical History

Student Name _____

Patient Initials _____ Room # _____ Admission Date _____

CODE Status _____ Today's Date _____ Age _____ Gender ____

Weight _____ Height _____

Braden Score _____ Diet _____ Activity _____

Religion _____ Allergies _____

Admitting Diagnoses/Chief Complaint

Assessment Data

Lab Values/Diagnostic Test Results

BMP

CBC

Misc Lab Values/Diagnostic Test Results

Treatments

Primary Nursing Diagnosis	Nursing Diagnosis 2	Nursing Diagnosis 3
Supporting Data	Supporting Data	Supporting Data
STG/NOC	STG/NOC	STG/NOC
Interventions/NIC with Rationale	Interventions/NIC with Rationale	Interventions/NIC with Rationale
Rationale Citation/EBP	Rationale Citation/EBP	Rationale Citation/EBP
Evaluation	Evaluation	Evaluation

ⓔ An interactive version of the Conceptual Care Map is on Evolve.

CASE STUDY 21

Alice Chung

Name/s _____ Date _____

Patient Assignment

A.C. is a 78-year-old Korean American female who fell in her home while doing laundry. She lives alone but had her mobile phone in her pocket. When she was unable to get herself off of the floor because of severe pain in her right hip, she called her daughter who lives nearby. Her daughter decided it was not a good idea to move A.C. so she dialed 911. A.C. is in the ED and x-rays show a fracture of the neck of the right femur. Open reduction internal fixation (ORIF) with pinning of the hip is planned for tomorrow morning.

A.C. is transferred to the orthopedic unit to wait for surgery. The ED nurse reports on the x-ray results and plan for surgery. The nurse states that A.C. is stable but in pain that she rates 7/10 after having received hydrocodone 5 mg/acetaminophen 325 mg PO 1 hour ago. A.C.'s daughter accompanies her to the unit.

Admitting Orders

Morphine 2 mg IV q 2 hr PRN for moderate to severe pain. NPO after midnight. Preoperative teaching regarding postoperative exercises, transfers, coughing and deep breathing, incentive spirometer. Bedrest. Maintain hip abduction with abductor pillow. IV 0.9% NS at 100 mL/hr.

1. After A.C. is transferred to your unit, what are your priority actions?

2. What questions will you ask A.C. and her daughter as you begin your assessment?

3. What is incentive spirometry?

4. What is the procedure for obtaining informed consent for the ORIF of the hip?

ASSESSMENT UPDATE

2100: A.C. is widowed and has another daughter who lives out of state. A.C. has been diagnosed with osteo-porosis but quit taking alendronate 4 years ago after having been on it for several years. She remembers leaning over to pick up the clothes basket tonight, and when she turned to leave the laundry room, she lost her balance. She does not think she hurt anything else, and she did not hit her head. She has never felt dizzy or lightheaded and has not fallen before tonight but has noticed that her balance is "not as good as it used to be." She takes multivitamins and calcium supplements at home and has an allergy to sulfa drugs. A.C. says that she enjoys music and reading and that she uses lavender essential oil on her wrist to relax at home. A.C. states that she has no religious affiliation. She does not have a living will and states that she has "been mean-ing to take care of that."

A.C. is a petite female: Height 157.5 cm (62 in), weight 48.6 kg (107 lb). VS: T 36.4° C (97.5° F), BP 116/78, P 78 and regular, R 20 and unlabored. O_2 saturation 96% on RA. Pain 7/10 in right hip. A&Ox4. PERRLA. Lungs clear. Apical pulse is 78 and regular. Abdomen is soft, and nontender. BS present in all four quadrants. Skin warm and dry. Braden score 20. Pedal pulses 2+ bilaterally. Normal strength and movement in both arms and left leg. Able to move toes on right foot. Normal sensation in all extremities. A.C. is in a supine position with an abductor pillow between her legs. IV infusing at 100 mL/hr in right hand through a 24-gauge catheter. No redness or swelling at site. A.C.'s adult daughter is in the room with her.

5. How is A.C.'s osteoporosis related to her fracture?

6. What preoperative teaching is important for you to begin tonight? Include step-by-step instructions.

7. What is the purpose of the abductor pillow?

8. Do you need written permission to discuss A.C.'s medical information with the out of state daughter if she calls, or with the daughter who is at the hospital, if A.C. is not present? Explain.

ASSESSMENT UPDATE

Day 2 1900: *You are starting your shift and are taking care of A.C. again. Her surgery was at 0900, and she returned to the unit at 1420.*

Postoperative orders: *Leave pressure dressing intact until changed by the surgeon. VS q 2 hr x 2 then q 4 hr. Clear liquid diet. Advance as tolerated. Physical therapy consult. Activity: up to chair with PT using walker and touchdown weight bearing. Cough and deep breathing exercises. Incentive Spirometer. Active or passive ROM exercises of arms and left leg. SCD to left leg when in bed.*

Morphine 2 mg IV q 2 hr PRN for moderate to severe pain. Docusate 100 mg PO q 12 hr; acetaminophen 325 mg 2 tablets PO q 6 hr PRN for mild to moderate pain; enoxaparin 40 mg subcut daily. IV 0.9% NS at 100 mL/hr. Convert IV to saline lock when patient is tolerating oral fluids. Ice pack to right hip q 2 hr for 20 min.

Report from day-shift nurse:

S: *A.C. has stable vital signs and is alert. There is no new drainage on her bandage. She has pain between 5-8/10 since she returned to the floor.*

B: *She is 10 hours postoperative ORIF of right hip with pinning. She has morphine 2 mg IV q 2 hr PRN for moderate to severe pain or acetaminophen 325 mg, 2 tablets PO q 6 hr PRN for mild to moderate pain.*

A: *A.C.'s pain was 8/10, and she was given IV morphine 2 mg at 1745. PT worked with her after she had morphine, and she sat on the side of the bed and stood beside the bed. A. C.'s pain level is currently 5/10.*

R: *Assess pain every 2 hours. Offer acetaminophen in addition to morphine. Use ice pack as ordered. Encourage deep breathing, relaxation, aromatherapy, and distraction as complimentary therapies.*

9. What postoperative complications is A.C. at risk for at this time? Two or more days from now?

10. Describe the step-by-step procedure for administering enoxaparin.

ASSESSMENT UPDATE

Day 2 1930: *VS: T 37.2° C (98.9° F), BP 116/70, P 78 and regular, R 18 and unlabored. O_2 saturation 97% on RA. Pain in right hip rated at 4/10, sharp and worse with movement. A&Ox4. PERRLA. Lungs clear. Apical pulse is 78 and regular. Abdomen is soft, nontender. BS present in all four quadrants. Skin warm and dry. Dressing on right hip covering surgical incision is dry with no visible drainage. Pedal pulses 2+ bilaterally. Moves toes on right foot and has sensation to sharp and dull objects in right leg. IV infusing in right hand. No redness or swelling at site. A.C.'s adult daughter is in the room with her. A.C. is sitting up in bed eating jello and tolerating clear liquids. She states that she is using the incentive spirometer often and the breathing exercises that were taught last night. A.C. would like to keep pain at 4/10 or under using medication, distraction, breathing, and aromatherapy. Her daughter brought her lavender oil from home.*

11. What are your top three nursing diagnoses with statements or patient problems for A.C. at this time?

12. What are some priority interventions for A.C. this evening?

13. Complete a CCM for Case Study 21 in this book or in the CCM Creator on Evolve for A.C. during her first evening postoperative. Be sure to record all of A.C.'s assessment data, medications, history, lab and test results, and treatments on the first page of the CCM. Use the three nursing diagnosis statements from question 11 to formulate an individualized plan of care. Use the Assessment Update on day 3 to evaluate the plan of care.

ASSESSMENT UPDATE

Day 3 1945: *VS: T 37.2° C (98.9° F), BP 116/70, P 78 and regular, R 18 and unlabored. O_2 saturation 97% on RA. Pain in right hip rated at 3/10, sharp and worse with movement. States that "the pain sure isn't as bad as it was yesterday. I've been reading and listening to music and doing that breathing thing. And the lavender scent helps to relax me" A&Ox4. PERRLA. Lungs clear. Apical pulse is 78 and regular. Abdomen is soft, nontender. BS present in all four quadrants. Skin warm and dry. Incision line dry, open to air, and well approximated. Staples intact. Pedal pulses 2+ bilaterally. Patient sitting up in chair with her feet flat on the floor. Able to transfer self from bed to chair and back using a walker as instructed by PT. States she had a bowel movement this morning for the first time in 2 ½ days.*

Additional Orders: *From this morning: D/C morphine and saline lock. Hydrocodone 5 mg/acetaminophen 325 mg, one tablet PO q 6 hr PRN for moderate to severe pain. Acetaminophen 325 mg, two tablets q 6 hr PO PRN for mild to moderate pain. Total acetaminophen not to exceed 3000 mg in 24 hours. Continue docusate 100 mg PO q 12 hr. Incision care: Leave open to air, cleanse with sterile NSS bid. Up in chair and bedside commode with elevated seat. Referral to rehab facility with possible discharge.*

14. What are the steps for cleansing an incision with staples?

15. What interventions will be important during hospitalization and when A.C. is discharged to a rehab facility?

Conceptual Care Map

Medications

Student Name _____

Patient Initials _____ Room # _____ Admission Date _____

CODE Status _____ Today's Date _____ Age _____ Gender _____

Weight _____ Height _____ Braden Score _____

Diet _____ Activity _____

Religion _____ Allergies _____

Lab Values/Diagnostic Test Results

BMP

CBC

Admitting Diagnoses/Chief Complaint

IV Sites/Fluids/Rate

Assessment Data

Misc Lab Values/Diagnostic Test Results

Past Medical/Surgical History

Treatments

Primary Nursing Diagnosis	Nursing Diagnosis 2	Nursing Diagnosis 3
Supporting Data	Supporting Data	Supporting Data
STG/NOC	STG/NOC	STG/NOC
Interventions/NIC with Rationale	Interventions/NIC with Rationale	Interventions/NIC with Rationale
Rationale Citation/EBP	Rationale Citation/EBP	Rationale Citation/EBP
Evaluation	Evaluation	Evaluation

ⓔ An interactive version of the Conceptual Care Map is on Evolve.

CASE STUDY

22

Karen Woodruff

Name/s _____ Date _____

Patient Assignment

K.W. is a 63-year-old female admitted to the hospital last night for hypovolemia and acute kidney injury (AKI). She has a 4-day history of nausea, vomiting, and diarrhea caused by gastroenteritis. When she came to the ED, she had been unable to keep oral fluids down and had not voided for over 12 hours. In the morning report, the night nurse tells you that K.W. has voided 200 mL during the 8-hour shift, which includes her urinalysis sample. She received 1000 mL of 0.9% NS in the ED. Her IV of 0.9% NS is now infusing at 100 mL/hr into her right hand. Intake for the night shift = 800 mL IV fluids. Output 200 mL. No vomiting or diarrhea. She is a bit confused, and her husband is at her bedside. She is a full code and has no allergies.

Day 1 0810 VS: T 37.2° C (99.0° F), BP 96/68, P 116 and regular, R 24 and slightly labored. O_2 saturation 95% on RA. Denies pain. Alert and oriented to person but confused about place, time, and situation. PERRLA. Lungs clear. Apical pulse is 114 and regular. BS hyperactive in all quadrants. Abdomen is firm, round, and nontender. States she still "feels a bit queasy but hasn't vomited lately." Skin warm and dry. Mucous membranes dry. Capillary refill >3 seconds. MAE. Pedal pulses 1+ bilaterally. IV infusing into right hand through a 22-gauge catheter. No redness or swelling at site. Height 165.1 cm (65 in). Weight 80 kg (176 lb). Braden score 19.

1. Which assessment data are of concern as you begin caring for K.W.?

2. To what do you attribute these findings?

3. Is this type of kidney injury reversible? How?

4. Will K.W. need dialysis? Include your rationale.

5. The PCP discusses the possibility of dialysis with K.W. and her husband, depending on her urine output and lab results over the next 24 hours. What is dialysis? What are the two types of dialysis? Explain briefly how each type works.

Admission Lab Results

BMP: Na 144 mEq/L, K 5.1 mEq/L, Cl 105 mEq/L, bicarb 18 mEq/L, BUN 45 mg/dL, creatinine 2.6 mg/dL, glucose 100 mg/dL; CBC: normal except Hct 49%; urinalysis: Normal except casts present, RBCs 6, WBCs 8, specific gravity 1.040. Estimated glomerular filtration rate (eGFR) 20 mL/min/1.73 m^2. (Lab results may vary by facility.)

6. Interpret K.W.'s lab results and place them in the Lab Values section of the CCM.

ASSESSMENT UPDATE

As you document K.W.'s morning assessment in the EHR, you review her chart and note that she has a repeat BMP ordered for tomorrow morning. She is on a clear liquid diet, and VS are ordered q 4 hr. She has orders for ondansetron 4 mg q 8 hr IV PRN for nausea and vomiting, which she last had at 0600. She has not had any diarrhea since she was in the ED. She is allowed up with assistance and is on strict I&O. Her religion is listed as Christian. Her past medical and surgical history is unremarkable. She has daily weights ordered.

7. What are your priority nursing diagnoses with statement, or patient problems, for K.W. today?

8. Write a goal statement for each nursing diagnosis or patient problem.

9. What interventions will be a priority for you as you care for K.W. today?

10. Complete a CCM for K.W. Use the priority nursing diagnostic statement or patient problem from Question 7 to formulate a plan of care for her.

11. As you complete your 8-hour shift from 0700 to 1500, you subtotal K.W.'s I&O for the day so far. She voided twice for a total of 240 mL. She took in oral fluids = 360 mL. She has had no vomiting or diarrhea. Remember to include her IV fluids for the shift. Calculate and interpret her fluid balance for the first 16 hours today. Does K. W. have a positive or negative intake-output balance so far today?

Day 1 I&O			
	Intake	Output	Intake-Output Balance
2300-0700			
0700-1500			
subtotal			
1500-2300			
Total for 24 hours			

12. What would you anticipate happening to her I&O balance over the next 48 hours? Give rationales.

ASSESSMENT UPDATE

Day 3 0745 VS: T 36.8° C (98.2° F), BP 108/74, P 92 and regular, R 20 and unlabored. O_2 saturation 97% on RA. Denies pain. A&Ox4. PERRLA. Lungs clear. Apical pulse is 94 and regular. BS normal in all four quadrants. Abdomen is firm, round, and nontender. Skin warm and dry. Mucous membranes moist. Capillary refill <2 seconds. MAE. Pedal pulses 2+ bilaterally. IV infusing into left hand at 80 mL/hr through a 22-gauge catheter. No redness or swelling at site. She is taking oral fluids and is now on a full liquid diet. She has not had any vomiting or diarrhea for 48 hours. She is allowed up ad lib.

I&O from Day 2			
	Intake	Output	Intake-Output Balance
2300-0700	900 mL	420 mL	
0700-1500	1160 mL	660 mL	
1500-2300	980 mL	720 mL	
Total for 24 hours	**3040 mL**	**1800 mL**	**+1240**

Day 3 BMP results: Na 143 mEq/L, K 5.0 mEq/L, Cl 104 mEq/L, bicarb 19 mEq/L, BUN 34 mg/dL, creatinine 1.9 mg/dL, glucose 90 mg/dL; eGFR 29 mL/min/1.73 m^2.

13. Interpret today's lab results.

14. What does her I&O from yesterday show you about her fluid balance?

15. What are your priorities as you care for her today? Give rationales.

ASSESSMENT UPDATE

Day 4 BMP results: *Normal except BUN 30 mg/dL, creatinine 1.6 mg/dL; eGFR 35 mL/min/1.73 m^2.*
   K.W.'s PCP saw her during morning rounds and discussed her lab values. She was told that her kidneys seemed to be improving every day and that there was no longer a need to consider dialysis. K.W. has continued to increase her oral intake and is now eating a regular diet. Her IV fluids are running at 50 mL/hr to continue stimulating kidney function. Tomorrow her lab results and I&O will be evaluated for possible discharge.

I&O from Day 3			
	Intake	Output	Intake-Output Balance
2300-0700	700 mL	480 mL	
0700-1500	820 mL	660 mL	
1500-2300	800 mL	620 mL	
Total for 24 hours	**2320 mL**	**1760 mL**	**+560**

16. As you begin planning for K.W.'s discharge, what patient education is the most important for her and her husband?

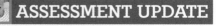

Day 5 BMP results: *Normal except BUN 24 mg/dL, creatinine 1.3 mg/dL; eGFR 45 mL/min/1.73 m².*

I&O from Day 4			
	Intake	Output	Intake-Output Balance
2300-0700	360 mL	350 mL	
0700-1500	1020 mL	960 mL	
1500-2300	780 mL	720 mL	
Total for 24 hours	**2160 mL**	**2030 mL**	**+130**

K.W. is discharged to home today. The PCP would like her to track her I&O for the next week, then be seen in the office in a week. She is dressed and ready to go home and her husband is at bedside.

17. Interpret her lab results from today (day 5) and I&O from yesterday (day 4).

18. K.W. asks whether she needs to measure her urine and what she eats. What teaching can be done to help the family measure I&O?

Medications

IV Sites/Fluids/Rate

Past Medical/Surgical History

Conceptual Care Map

Student Name_____

Patient Initials _____ Room # _____ Admission Date _____

CODE Status _____ Today's Date _____ Age_____ Gender _____

Weight _____ Height _____ Braden Score _____

Diet _____ Activity _____

Religion _____ Allergies _____

Admitting Diagnoses/Chief Complaint

Assessment Data

Lab Values/Diagnostic Test Results

BMP

CBC

Misc Lab Values/Diagnostic Test Results

Treatments

Primary Nursing Diagnosis	Nursing Diagnosis 2	Nursing Diagnosis 3
Supporting Data	Supporting Data	Supporting Data
STG/NOC	STG/NOC	STG/NOC
Interventions/NIC with Rationale	Interventions/NIC with Rationale	Interventions/NIC with Rationale
Rationale Citation/EBP	Rationale Citation/EBP	Rationale Citation/EBP
Evaluation	Evaluation	Evaluation

e An interactive version of the Conceptual Care Map is on Evolve.

23

Mark Summerfield

Name/s _____ Date _____

Patient Assignment

M.S. is a 64-year-old male who had a colon resection and temporary colostomy 3 days ago for colon cancer. The surgical report indicates that the tumor was through all layers of the descending colon, with no obvious lymph nodes or other organs involved. The tumor was removed along with 13 cm of the colon in the middle part of the descending colon. Both ends were brought through the abdominal wall creating a double-barreled stoma on the mid-left side of the abdomen. Several lymph nodes were removed for biopsy.

M.S.'s history states that he had his first colonoscopy recently after noticing blood in his stools. The tumor was discovered during the colonoscopy. M.S. has hypertension, has smoked two packs per day (ppd) of cigarettes for 45 years, and drinks two or three beers most evenings. His diet consists of mostly meats, potatoes, burgers and steaks on the grill, and sandwiches for lunch. He states his religion as Lutheran. M.S. is 177.8 cm (70 in) tall and weighs 96.4 kg (212 lb). He does not know of any family history of colon cancer, but his brother had some polyps removed a few years ago. He has a peanut allergy and has full code status.

1. What are the recommendations and screening schedule for colon cancer?

2. What risk factors did M.S. have for developing colon cancer?

3. What is a double-barrel colostomy?

4. What kind of stool will drain from M.S.'s colostomy?

5. What other types of bowel diversion ostomies are there? Where will the stoma be placed? What type of stool will likely drain from each?

ASSESSMENT UPDATE

Postoperative day 3: 0830 VS: T 36.4° C (97.5° F), BP 136/82, P 80 and regular, R 24 and unlabored. O_2 saturation 92% on RA. A&Ox4, PERRLA. Pain 2/10 near his incision. Lungs: wheezing in all lung fields on auscultation. Apical pulse is 80 and regular. Abdomen is soft, round, and tender. Bowel sounds present in all four quadrants. Two stomas are beefy red in color and raised 1.2 cm above the surrounding skin. Colostomy bag is in place over the upper stoma. The lower stoma is covered with gauze. Thirteen cm midline incision is dry, pink and well approximated with staples intact. Incision is open to air. One cm round healing area to the right of the incision where Jackson-Pratt (JP) drain was removed is dry and closed. Skin warm and dry. Braden score 22. MAE. Pedal pulses 2+ bilaterally.

M.S. is sitting up in bed. His wife is sitting next to the bed. He states that he walked to the bathroom this morning with his wife by his side. He states that the pain is not as bad as it was for a couple of days. He would like to try taking only acetaminophen today for pain and had two tablets at 0600, which he says decreased his pain. He refused docusate this morning stating that he did not plan to take oxycodone today.

Current Orders: Lisinopril 10 mg PO once daily. Oxycodone 5 mg PO q 4 hr PRN for moderate to severe pain. Docusate 100 mg PO q 12 h if taking oxycodone; acetaminophen 500 mg tabs, two tabs PO q 6 hr PRN for mild to moderate pain; enoxaparin 80 mg subcut daily. SCDs while in bed. Consult Wound Ostomy Continence Nurse (WOCN) for colostomy teaching and acquisition of supplies for ostomy. VS and stoma assessment q 4 hr. Incision care: leave open to air, and cleanse with sterile normal saline solution (NSS) tid. Up with assistance. Adult general diet.

6. A JP drain was removed yesterday. Label the drains pictured below and briefly describe how each works.

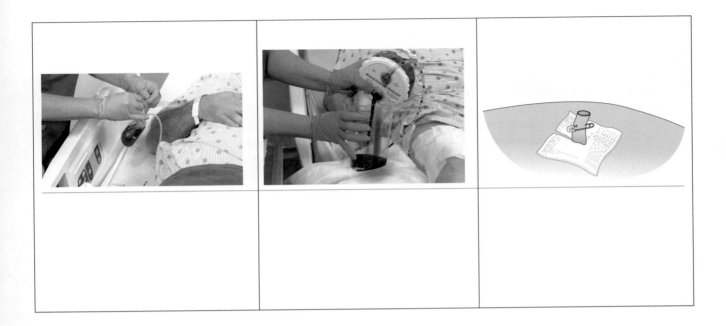

7. M.S.'s colostomy appliance is coming loose on the upper stoma. List at least three important reasons to change an ostomy pouch system when it is loose.

8. Make a list of the supplies that are needed to change the two-piece ostomy pouch system.

9. List the steps necessary to change the appliance.

10. Document a sample narrative note about the colostomy appliance change procedure. Include important assessment findings noted during the colostomy change.

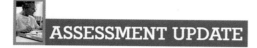

ASSESSMENT UPDATE

Postoperative day 3, 1100: During ostomy care, M.S. shares that he is "disgusted" about having a colostomy. He refuses to watch the procedure and states that he does not know how he is going to do this at home. His wife is at bedside and says that she wants to learn so that she can help him. M.S. agrees to let her watch the procedure. During the procedure, M.S. turns his head away. His wife asks several appropriate questions as each step is explained and questions answered.

11. What can you do to help M.S. begin to accept his condition?

12. How does patient with a colostomy control gas and odor?

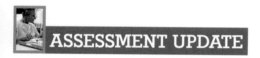

ASSESSMENT UPDATE

Postoperative day 3, 1110: The oncologist makes rounds and recommends chemotherapy even though the cancerous cells had not spread to the adjoining structures or lymph nodes. The oncologist outlines the options, risks, and benefits of having chemo and tells M.S. that the decision is his. M.S. states that he is anxious about undergoing chemotherapy, especially since he has so much to deal with right now. He is concerned about healing from surgery, the colostomy, missing work, finances, and placing additional burdens on his wife who "has health problems of her own." He says, "I just don't know what to do."

The WOCN has written a teaching plan for M.S. and his wife. It includes what to expect from the colostomy, how to care for a colostomy, what foods to avoid, and what signs and symptoms may indicate a problem. A booklet and a video were given to the couple and teaching is in process.

13. What is the nurse's role in helping M.S. make a decision about chemotherapy?

14. With which other members of the health care team might you collaborate for M.S.'s care, teaching, and discharge planning? What is the role of each member of the team?

15. Using all of the assessment data, make a list of nursing diagnoses or patient problems that might be included in M.S.'s care plan.

16. What discharge teaching is important for M.S. and his wife before discharge to home?

17. Complete a CCM for Case Study 23 in this book or in the CCM Creator on Evolve for M.S. Enter all assessment data into the CCM, and use three of the nursing diagnoses or patient problems that are listed in Question 15 to formulate a care plan for M.S.

Conceptual Care Map

Medications

IV Sites/Fluids/Rate

Past Medical/Surgical History

Student Name _____

Patient Initials _____ Room # _____ Admission Date _____

CODE Status _____ Today's Date _____ Age _____ Gender _____

Weight _____ Height _____ Braden Score _____

Diet _____ Activity _____

Religion _____ Allergies _____

Admitting Diagnoses/Chief Complaint

Assessment Data

Lab Values/Diagnostic Test Results

BMP

CBC

Misc Lab Values/Diagnostic Test Results

Treatments

Primary Nursing Diagnosis	Nursing Diagnosis 2	Nursing Diagnosis 3
Supporting Data	Supporting Data	Supporting Data
STG/NOC	STG/NOC	STG/NOC
Interventions/NIC with Rationale	Interventions/NIC with Rationale	Interventions/NIC with Rationale
Rationale Citation/EBP	Rationale Citation/EBP	Rationale Citation/EBP
Evaluation	Evaluation	Evaluation

ⓔ An interactive version of the Conceptual Care Map is on Evolve.

CASE STUDY

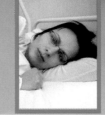

24

Sarah Laurent

Name/s _____   Date _____

Patient Assignment

S.L. is a 35-year-old female admitted to the hospital today with severe abdominal pain, liquid stools 7 to 10 times daily, and blood in her stool. She has an 8-year history of Crohn's disease. S.L.'s symptoms have worsened over the last week. She had taken prednisone for several months and was weaned off of the medication a couple of months ago.

Initial Assessment

1400 VS: T 38.2° C (100.8° F), BP 106/68, P 94 and regular, R 24 and unlabored. O_2 saturation 94% on RA. Pain 7/10 in right lower abdominal quadrant that is intermittent. A&O×4, PERRLA. Lungs clear. Apical pulse is 94 and regular. BS hyperactive in all quadrants. Abdomen is firm, distended, and tender over the right lower quadrant, no masses palpable. Skin warm, pale, and dry. Capillary refill <2 seconds. MAE. Pedal pulses 2+ bilaterally. IV infusing into left forearm through a 22-gauge catheter. No redness or swelling at site. Height 170.2 cm (67 in). Weight 52.7 kg (116 lb). Braden score 22.

Admission Orders

— check for metabolism

CBC; BMP; Fe; prealbumin; stool culture; guaiac stools; I&O including number and character of stools; daily weights; up with assistance; NPO, bowel rest; IV D_5W, infuse at 80 mL/hr; IV methylprednisolone 80 mg in 50 mL D_5W q 6 hr, infuse over 15 minutes; blood glucose fingerstick q 8 hr; acetaminophen 500 mg, two tablets q 6 hr PO PRN for pain. Full code

1. What assessment findings indicate an exacerbation of S.L.'s Crohn's disease?

2. What is the rationale behind her NPO status?

3. Which assessment questions are important to ask S.L.?

4. What rate will you set on the IV infusion pump to administer the methylprednisolone on time?

5. What is the rationale behind ordering fingerstick blood glucose levels q 8 hr?

ASSESSMENT UPDATE

S.L. has had flare-ups once or twice a year since diagnosis. She cannot think of anything that precipitated this flare-up. She lives with her husband and children ages 9 and 11. They are originally from out of state, so most of the friends she has are either neighbors or church or work friends. The family attends a United Methodist church. S.L. is an occupational therapist at a skilled nursing/rehabilitation facility. She is concerned about missing work because there is no one to cover for her right now. She is also concerned about her children's activities and transportation while she is hospitalized. The only new symptom that S.L. has noticed lately is that she gets "light-headed" when she stands up too quickly. S.L. states that the "frequent liquid stools along with the cramping are making me feel so tired and ill. I have no energy anymore, so I haven't been doing my walking for exercise." The only medications she has been taking at home are calcium supplements.

S.L. has followed a low-residue diet for years, although she admits to "cheating" a bit lately. She describes her abdominal pain as "coming and going like waves of pain." She says that she has lost 6 or 7 lb recently because her stomach hurt so much that she did not have an appetite. She states that she has no allergies

Lab Results: BMP: Na 134 mEq/L, K 3.3 mEq/L, Cl 92 mEq/L, bicarb 18 mEq/L, BUN 20 mg/dL, creatinine 1.2 mg/dL, Glucose 120 mg/dL; CBC: WBC 12,000/mm^3, Hgb 9 g/dL, Hct 31%, platelets 400,000 x 10^9/L; Fe 54 mcg/dL; prealbumin 18 mg/dL. Stool guaiac tests: positive. Stool cultures pending. (Lab results may vary by facility.)

6. Place the lab results in the CCM for S.L. Be sure to give the normal ranges for all abnormal lab values and interpret the abnormal values by relating them to the information about S.L.

7. What might be causing her symptom of lightheadedness?

8. Write three nursing diagnosis statements or patient problems for S.L. Prioritize the statements in order of urgency and importance.

9. Give rationales as to why you ranked the nursing diagnoses in a particular order.

10. List at least five other nursing diagnosis labels or patient problems for S.L.

11. Which precautions will you put into place for S.L.? Explain your rationale and what these precautions entail.

12. Which aspects of care can be delegated to the UAP?

13. What instructions should you give to S.L. and the UAP regarding her perineal care?

1800 VS: T 37.0° C (98.6° F), BP 108/70, P 84 and regular, R 20 and unlabored. O_2 saturation 96% on RA. BS hyperactive in all four quadrants. Has had one dose of acetaminophen at 1420 for pain 7/10 that was intermittent. Pain 4/10 in right lower abdominal quadrant. States that the pain is not as intense and that she has only had one loose stool since she came to the floor. Assessment otherwise unchanged.

New Orders: *Change IV solution to lactated ringers. Infuse at 80 mL/hr. Dietitian consult. Referral to counseling for relaxation and stress management. Repeat BMP tomorrow morning.*

14. What is the rationale behind the change in IV solutions?

15. In collaboration with the dietitian, what dietary instructions will be important for S.L. when she is discharged?

16. Discuss with S.L. how she might prevent flare-ups in the future.

17. What medication will S.L. most likely be discharged on? What teaching should you provide concerning the medication?

18. Complete a CCM for Case Study 24 in this book or in the CCM Creator on Evolve for S.L. Use the priority nursing diagnostic statements or patient problems from question 8, and formulate a plan of care for S.L.

Medications

Conceptual Care Map

Student Name_____

Patient Initials _____ Room # _____ Admission Date _____

Code Status _____ Today's Date _____ Age_____ Gender _____

Weight _____ Height _____ Braden Score _____

Diet _____ Activity _____

Religion _____ Allergies _____

Lab Values/Diagnostic Test Results

BMP

CBC

Admitting Diagnoses/Chief Complaint

Assessment Data

IV Sites/Fluids/Rate

Misc Lab Values/Diagnostic Test Results

Past Medical/Surgical History

Treatments

Primary Nursing Diagnosis	Nursing Diagnosis #2	Nursing Diagnosis #3
Supporting Data	Supporting Data	Supporting Data
STG/NOC	STG/NOC	STG/NOC
Interventions/NIC with Rationale	Interventions/NIC with Rationale	Interventions/NIC with Rationale
Rationale Citation/EBP	Rationale Citation/EBP	Rationale Citation/EBP
Evaluation	Evaluation	Evaluation

ⓔ An interactive version of the Conceptual Care Map is on Evolve.

CASE STUDY

25

Broderick Winston

Name/s _____   Date _____

Patient Assignment

B.W. is an 84-year-old, 180.3 cm (71 in), 76.4 kg (168 lb) retired teacher who presented to the ED 8 days ago with clinical manifestations of a cerebrovascular accident (CVA), including severe aphasia, that had begun 2 hours earlier. Following a stat CT scan, he was treated with IV alteplase and stabilized. Since being admitted to the nursing unit, he has started rehabilitation and is preparing for transfer to a rehab facility in the community in which he lives. B.W. has a history of HTN, smoking (20+ years, quit 40 years ago), appendectomy 43 years ago, R hip replacement 5 years ago. He is a recent widower, having been married for 63 years. He lives alone. His children all live out of state. B.W. is a full code, Baptist, with allergies to ciprofloxacin and iodine.

Initial Assessment

0700 VS: T 36.8° C (98.2°F), BP 167/88, P 92 and regular, R 18 and unlabored. O_2 sat 95% on RA. Occasional wincing with movement. Reports "stinging" pain 2–3/10 in R hip, A&O×3–4. Slow speech. Follows most directions given time. Slight right facial droop, right upper and lower extremity weakness. Lungs are diminished in the bases, no cough present. Apical pulse 92 bpm. Abdomen is slightly distended with normal BS on the left and decreased BS in both right upper and lower quadrants. Urine is clear and pale yellow. Experiences some difficulty voiding. Dorsalis pedis pulses are 2+ bilaterally. Capillary refill <2 seconds. 20 g saline lock left forearm (LFA). Braden score is 20.

Admission Orders

Treatments: VS q 4 hr including neuro checks, falls precautions, ambulate with assistance, NPO until swallow evaluation, PT, OT, I&O, bladder scan and straight cath PRN, knee-high antiembolic stockings, SCDs, BMP, CBC, aPTT, PT/INR daily.

Medications: 1000 mL D_5W @ 125 mL/hr, heparin 5,000 units subcut q 8 hr, metoprolol 100 mg PO bid, lisinopril 20 mg PO daily, milk of magnesia 30 mL PO PRN, acetaminophen 650 mg PO PRN.

1. Identify the two major types of CVA based on etiology.

2. Briefly explain the purpose of a stat CT scan when someone presents to the ED with signs and symptoms of a CVA.

3. What is the classification of alteplase? Which of the major two types of CVA is it used to treat? Since B.W. was treated with alteplase, what type of CVA did he have?

4. From B.W.'s initial assessment findings, identify the side of the brain in which his CVA occurred.

5. Complete the chart below by listing clinical manifestations of CVAs occurring in the right and left sides of the brain.

Right Brain CVA	Left Brain CVA

6. Define the terms *aphasia* and *aphagia*. Provide an idea of how you could help a patient or student to remember the difference.

7. Identify the two major types of aphasia, and provide a brief explanation of each.

8. List a minimum of 12 risk factors for CVA. Highlight those that are modifiable either through life-style changes or medical intervention.

9. Begin B.W.'s patient-centered plan of care by filling in his admission information, initial assessment findings, treatment, and medication orders in the CCM.

10. To complete a thorough neurologic assessment, you need to check B.W.'s cranial nerves. Of particular interest are cranial nerves II, VII, and X. In the table below, (1) name these three cranial nerves, (2) share how to assess each one and, (3) list one or two symptoms associated with damage to each of the nerves.

Cranial Nerve Number	Cranial Nerve Name	Assessment	Symptoms Associated with Damage
II			
VII			
X			

11. What aspects of B.W.'s assessment can be delegated to unlicensed assistive personnel (UAP)? What are the responsibilities of the registered nurse (RN) in delegation?

ASSESSMENT UPDATE

1100 VS: T 34.6° C (94.3°F), BP 146/78, P 74 and regular, R 18 and unlabored. O$_2$ sat 97% on RA. Continued R hip pain of 2/10. A&Ox3 -4. Neuro status unchanged. Slow speech. Passed swallow test with some difficulty. Diet advanced to low sodium with thickened liquids, as needed. DC IV fluids. Convert access to saline lock. Lungs clear in upper lobes, diminished bilaterally in lower lobes. Apical pulse 74 bpm. Abdomen soft, BSx4. Urinating without difficulty. Pedal pulses 2+ bilaterally, no edema. Ambulating with PT assistance and quad cane. Working with OT bid. Patient frustration and discouragement with slow progress documented by both PT and OT. Scheduled for discharge in A.M. to Whispering Pines Rehabilitation Center.

Current lab results:

BMP	CBC
Na$^+$ 145 mEq/L	*WBC 7 × 10^9/L*
K$^+$ 4.3 mEq/L	*Hgb 15.5 g/dL*
Cl$^-$ 108 mEq/L	*Hct 42.8%*
CO$_2$ 25 mEq/L	*Plt 307 × 10^9/L*
BUN 14 mg/dL	
Creatinine 0.84 mg/dL	*aPTT-52 seconds*
BS 103 mg/dL	*PT/INR -12.8/1.2*

12. Note the temperature reading (T 34.6° C [94.3°F]) that the UAP reported for B.W. What action should the RN request the UAP to take as a result of this finding? If you had been assessing B.W.'s vital signs initially and gotten that temperature reading, what initial action would have been appropriate for you to take?

13. Although B.W. is able to swallow, the treatment orders include thickened liquids PRN. What is the rationale for thickening some of his liquid intake? Explain the procedure for thickening liquids for patients with difficulty swallowing.

14. What is your analysis of B.W.'s current aPTT and PT/INR findings? Why are these lab tests being ordered for him? Include your specific analysis on B.W.'s CCM.

15. Briefly explain the role of speech, physical, and occupational therapy in B.W.'s care.

16. As the RN for B.W., you are responsible for coordinating his care in preparation for discharge. In addition to speech therapy, PT, and OT, what members of the health care team are important to making B.W.'s transition to a rehabilitation facility as smooth as possible?

17. Identify three priority nursing diagnoses for B.W. on his eighth hospital day. Complete your CCM to address these concerns.

Conceptual Care Map

Medications

IV Sites/Fluids/Rate

Past Medical/Surgical History

Student Name_____

Patient Initials _____ Room # _____ Admission Date _____

CODE Status _____ Today's Date _____ Age_____ Gender _____

Weight _____ Height _____ Braden Score _____

Diet _____ Activity _____

Religion _____ Allergies _____

Admitting Diagnoses/Chief Complaint

Assessment Data

Lab Values/Diagnostic Test Results

BMP

CBC

Misc Lab Values/Diagnostic Test Results

Treatments

Primary Nursing Diagnosis	Nursing Diagnosis 2	Nursing Diagnosis 3
Supporting Data	Supporting Data	Supporting Data
STG/NOC	STG/NOC	STG/NOC
Interventions/NIC with Rationale	Interventions/NIC with Rationale	Interventions/NIC with Rationale
Rationale Citation/EBP	Rationale Citation/EBP	Rationale Citation/EBP
Evaluation	Evaluation	Evaluation

ⓔ An interactive version of the Conceptual Care Map is on Evolve.

CASE STUDY

26

Caleb Nguyen

Name/s _____ Date _____

Patient Assignment

C.N. is a 28-year-old, admitted to your unit overnight with cellulitis of the right leg. C.N. was hiking the Appalachian Trail 3 days ago and was bitten by an unknown insect. He reports that his leg became red and swollen almost immediately and itched really badly. He has been taking diphenhydramine occasionally but realized he needed help when he developed a fever. He is a full code, is allergic to cephalosporin drugs and peanuts, and has a Braden score of 21. C.N. identifies himself as Catholic and is ordered an adult general diet. He is on bed rest with bathroom privileges.

Initial Assessment

0740 VS T 39.4° C (102.9° F), BP 126/64, P 54 and regular, R 16 and unlabored. O_2 sat 100% on RA. Aching, burning pain of 3/10 in right leg. Experiencing chills and diaphoresis with his fever. A&O×4. Lungs clear bilaterally in all lobes. Apical pulse 54 bpm. Abdomen is soft, flat with BSx4. Urine clear, light yellow. LBM yesterday. 1+ pitting edema R leg below knee to ankle. R posterior tibial pulse 1+, L 2+. Capillary refill R foot >2 seconds, L foot <2 seconds. 22-gauge saline lock LH.

1. What is the etiology of cellulitis and when does it typically occur?

2. List the most common clinical manifestations of cellulitis.

3. C.N.'s Braden score is 21. Name the six categories that are assessed by the Braden scale. Identify the two categories in which he would achieve lower than a maximum score and provide a rationale for your answer.

4. What is the most serious potential complication of cellulitis?

5. What is the classification of diphenhydramine and how would it help a person who initially appears to have an allergic reaction to an insect bite?

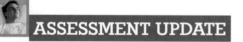

ASSESSMENT UPDATE

After morning rounds by C.N.'s PCP, his orders are revised to include VS q 8 hr, R leg wet→dry dressing changes bid, elevate R leg 30 degrees while in bed, falls precautions, I&O, CBC daily, knee-high antiembolic stocking L leg, sequential compression device (SCD) L leg, heparin 5000 units subcut bid, cefazolin 500 mg in 50 mL D$_5$W IV q 6 hr, acetaminophen 650 mg PO PRN.

6. You need to initiate the knee-high antiembolic stocking order for C.N. Explain the rationale for ordering an antiembolic stocking for C.N.'s left leg and describe the procedure for measuring and applying this type of stocking.

7. Explain the procedure for applying SCDs. Include in your explanation examples of when SCDs should be applied and removed from a patient while they have them ordered.

8. Observe the cellulitis in the photo provided. What is the purpose of the markings at the edge of the reddened area? Provide an explanation of what documentation of a focused wound assessment would include.

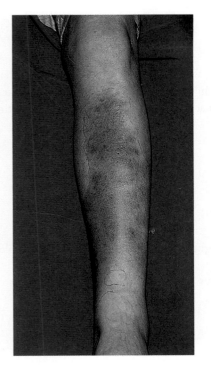

9. Describe the purpose of a wet→dry dressing and the procedure for applying it to C.N.'s leg.

ASSESSMENT UPDATE

C.N.'s CBC results are below:

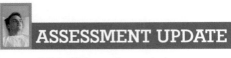

10. Enter all of C.N.'s assessment data, orders, and lab results into the CCM. Analyze the lab results and provide thorough medication information as required to complete your CCM.

11. C.N. refuses to take the heparin 5000 units subcutaneously when you enter the room to give him his first dose. Briefly provide the explanation you would give to C.N. regarding the importance of his taking the injection.

12. After you discuss the importance of heparin and how it is given, C.N. tells you that he just does not like needles and agrees to have the heparin injection. What action would you take if C.N. had continued to refuse the heparin even after you had provided him with more information?

13. What three checks (in addition to the six rights of administration) must be completed before giving patient medications?

14. What error do you note in C.N.'s current medication orders? What action do you as his nurse take?

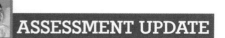
ASSESSMENT UPDATE

1500 VS T 39.5° C (103.1° F), BP 132/74, P 62 and regular, R 18 and unlabored. O$_2$ sat 99% on RA. Pain 4/10 R leg. Medication order DC cefazolin, clindamycin 600 mg in 50 mL q 6 hr IV.

15. At what rate (mL/hr) will you set the infusion pump to run the clindamycin over 20 minutes?

16. In addition to starting treatment with antibiotics, what additional medication should you give to C.N. in response to his latest vital signs?

17. Add the latest assessment update information to C.N.'s CCM and complete his patient-centered plan of care with three nursing diagnoses.

Conceptual Care Map

Medications

IV Sites/Fluids/Rate

Past Medical/Surgical History

Student Name_____

Patient Initials _____ Room # _____ Admission Date _____

CODE Status _____ Today's Date _____ Age_____ Gender _____

Weight _____ Height _____ Braden Score _____

Diet _____ Activity _____

Religion _____ Allergies _____

Admitting Diagnoses/Chief Complaint

Assessment Data

Lab Values/Diagnostic Test Results

BMP

CBC

Misc Lab Values/Diagnostic Test Results

Treatments

Primary Nursing Diagnosis	Nursing Diagnosis 2	Nursing Diagnosis 3
Supporting Data	Supporting Data	Supporting Data
STG/NOC	STG/NOC	STG/NOC
Interventions/NIC with Rationale	Interventions/NIC with Rationale	Interventions/NIC with Rationale
Rationale Citation/EBP	Rationale Citation/EBP	Rationale Citation/EBP
Evaluation	Evaluation	Evaluation

ⓔ An interactive version of the Conceptual Care Map is on Evolve.

CASE STUDY

27

Edward Moore

Name/s _____ **Date** _____

Patient Assignment

E.M. is a 69-year-old African American male. He is being seen on a Tuesday at the nephrologist's office for a routine appointment. He started hemodialysis (HD) three times per week (Monday, Wednesday, and Friday) 2 months ago. E.M. is awaiting kidney transplantation. He is a married father of three grown children and has five grandchildren ages 3 through 17. His relatives are currently being tested as possible donors, and he has been placed on the transplant list. E.M. is on a no added salt (NAS) diet, 1500 mL/day fluid restriction, and activity as tolerated.

E.M.'s past medical, surgical, social, and family history includes:

- No known drug allergies
- Married for 45 years, retired
- Lifelong member of the American Methodist Episcopal Church
- Hypertension (HTN) for 26 years, controlled with furosemide and diltiazem
- Type 2 diabetes mellitus (DM) for 22 years, controlled with glyburide and diet. HbA_{1C} 6.8%
- Chronic kidney disease (CKD) for 4 years
- Arteriovenous fistula (AVF) placed 4 months ago in left forearm
- End-stage kidney disease (ESKD) for 2 months
- Father died at age 64 of ESKD and also had type 2 DM, CAD, and HTN
- Mother is 91 and has age-related macular degeneration and Alzheimer's disease
- Wife, age 68, had a hysterectomy 10 years ago and has diverticulitis
- Brother died at age 71 of complications from type 2 DM
- Brother, age 67, no major medical problems
- Sister, age 63, no major medical problems
- Two daughters, age 35 no major medical problems, and age 42, has type 2 DM
- One son, age 38, no major medical problems

1. What risk factors did E.M. have for developing CKD?

2. Of the relatives listed, who is a possible kidney donor based on the information provided?

3. What is the AVF that E.M. had placed 4 months ago?

4. Briefly explain HD.

5. Since E.M. is undergoing HD and has an AVF, how will you assess his AVF? What signs and symptoms might indicate that his AVF has failed?

ASSESSMENT UPDATE

Tuesday 1530 VS: T 36.2° C (97.2° F), BP 136/82, P 86 and regular, R 20. O_2 saturation 97% on RA. Denies pain. A&O×4. PERRLA. Lungs clear. Apical pulse is 84 and regular. BS present in four quadrants. Abdomen is soft and nontender. Skin warm and dry. Capillary refill <2 seconds. MAE. 1+ pitting edema bilaterally in lower extremities. Pedal pulses 2+ bilaterally. Right radial pulse 2+. Left forearm, thrill palpated and bruit heard over AVF. Height 180.4 cm (71 in). Weight 97.7 kg (215 lb). BMI 30.0.

E.M. states that he is feeling better since starting dialysis. But he states that "it does take a big chunk of my time." He states that he is "tired and needs to take a nap most days." His wife accompanied him to the appointment and usually goes with him to dialysis. He has a list of questions for the nephrologist about kidney transplantation both as a recipient and about the donor. States he is "anxious about the surgery both for myself and for whoever is the donor but is willing to do whatever it takes to stay healthy enough for the surgery. "He urinates approximately 400 to 500 mL/day. While reviewing his EHR, you notice that his postdialysis weight yesterday morning was 96.3 kg (211.8 lb), BMI 29.5.

E.M.'s current medications are:

- *Furosemide 80 mg PO every morning*
- *Diltiazem 60 mg PO bid*
- *Glyburide 10 mg PO daily*
- *Sodium ferric gluconate complex 10 mL IV with each HD treatment*

6. What can you tell E.M. about his BMI?

7. The dietitian has outlined a diet for E.W. to follow. What basic guidelines would you anticipate for E.M.'s diet? Consider his need to lose weight, his HD, and his chronic illnesses.

8. What are the classifications and rationales behind each of E.M.'s medications? Place this information in the CCM for E.M.

9. Explain how E.M. was diagnosed with ESKD even though he is still producing urine.

10. List at least three nursing diagnoses with statements or patient problems that are a priority for E.M. at this office visit.

11. Complete a CCM for Case Study 27 in this book or in the CCM Creator on Evolve for E.M. Use the three nursing diagnostic statement or patient problem from the previous question, and formulate a plan of care for him. Include all data so far from this office visit. Evaluate your plan of care based on today's office visit.

ASSESSMENT UPDATE

The nephrologist answers E.M.'s questions by explaining organ donation and procurement policies to him and his wife. He tells them that the best option for transplant would be a live donor kidney from a family member. If that is not possible, organ donation is governed by Organ Procurement and Transplantation Network policies under contract to the US Department of Health and Human Services. Decisions about who receives available organs are made using medical information and logistic considerations. In general, blood type, size of the patient, time spent awaiting transplant, and the distance the donor organ would have to travel are considered. Other factors such as medical urgency of the recipient, the match between donor and recipient, and whether the recipient is a child or an adult are taken into account (From United Network for Organ Sharing. 2015. Frequently asked questions. https://www.unos.org/transplantation/faqs/#age).

The nephrologist also shares that two of E.M.'s relatives who volunteered to be tested as donors are potential matches. E.M. is cautioned that further testing and evaluations need to be done before it is known if they are able to be donors. He offers counseling for E.M. and his wife to deal with the psychological aspects of being an organ recipient.

12. What sort of testing is involved for live donors?

13. E.M. asks what he can do to prepare for surgery in case he is lucky enough to find a live donor. What instructions will he be given?

14. How is the kidney transplanted into the recipient during surgery? What is the usual postoperative course for kidney transplant recipients?

15. What type of surgical procedure is used to remove the donor kidney? What is the usual postoperative course for kidney transplant donors?

ASSESSMENT UPDATE

One month later: The nephrologist has determined that E.M.'s 67-year-old brother and 38-year-old son are both ABO compatible with E.M. After further testing, it is decided that his son is the best candidate for donating a kidney. E.M.'s son has shared this news with him.

At E.M.'s nephrology appointment, the doctor discusses the risks and benefits transplant surgery, and postoperative care. The surgery is planned for next month.

16. What are some of the risks of kidney transplant surgery for both the donor and the recipient?

17. If rejection does not occur, what are the benefits of kidney transplant surgery?

Conceptual Care Map

Medications

IV Sites/Fluids/Rate

Past Medical/Surgical History

Student Name_____

Patient Initials _____ Room # _____ Admission Date _____

CODE Status _____ Today's Date _____ Age_____ Gender _____

Weight _____ Height _____ Braden Score _____

Diet _____ Activity _____

Religion _____ Allergies _____

Admitting Diagnoses/Chief Complaint

Assessment Data

Lab Values/Diagnostic Test Results

BMP

CBC

Misc Lab Values/Diagnostic Test Results

Treatments

Primary Nursing Diagnosis	Nursing Diagnosis 2	Nursing Diagnosis 3
Supporting Data	Supporting Data	Supporting Data
STG/NOC	STG/NOC	STG/NOC
Interventions/NIC with Rationale	Interventions/NIC with Rationale	Interventions/NIC with Rationale
Rationale Citation/EBP	Rationale Citation/EBP	Rationale Citation/EBP
Evaluation	Evaluation	Evaluation

ⓔ An interactive version of the Conceptual Care Map is on Evolve.

CASE STUDY

28 Taylor Collins

Name/s _____ Date _____

Patient Assignment

T.C., a 34-year-old type I diabetic, is being transferred to your nursing unit from the intensive care unit (ICU). Report from the ICU nurse indicates that T.C.'s blood sugar is now 72 after having been 438 upon arrival to the unit 2 days ago from the emergency department (ED). T.C. is a brittle diabetic who is hospitalized at least five times a year because of diabetic ketoacidosis (DKA) or diabetic hypoglycemia. She is experiencing neuropathy in her lower extremities and vision problems. She has a history of appendectomy 15 years ago and recreational marijuana use. T.C. is a full code, with allergies to oxycodone, codeine, meperidine, and eggs. Her Braden score is 23, and her diet and activity orders are ADA 2200 and up ad lib, respectively. T.C. is 167.6 cm (66 in) tall and weighs 47.6 kg (105 lb). She was diagnosed with diabetes at age 10.

Initial Assessment

0730 VS T 36.4° C (97.5°F), BP 122/58, P 78 and regular, R 20 and unlabored. O_2 sat 98% on RA. Pain 4-5/10 in both legs and feet, accompanied by numbness and tingling; Pain described as "prickling" by patient. A&O×4. Lungs clear bilaterally in all lobes. Apical pulse 78 bpm. Abdomen is soft, flat with BS×4. Urine clear, light yellow. MAE denies constipation or diarrhea. Capillary refill <3 seconds in hands, >3 seconds in feet, pedal pulses 1+ bilaterally, no edema. 22-gauge intracath LH with $D_5\frac{1}{2}$ NS infusing at 150 mL/hr. IV site without redness or swelling; dressing signed and dated.

1. Briefly describe the difference between type I and type II diabetes.

2. Classic symptoms at the onset of type I diabetes are described as the three Ps. List the three Ps, and explain each one.

3. Define and discuss the difference between DKA and diabetic hypoglycemia. Which was T.C. experiencing when she arrived at the ED?

4. List possible clinical manifestations associated with DKA and diabetic hypoglycemia in the table provided.

DKA	DIABETIC HYPOGLYCEMIA

5. What lab values would be most important to monitor for patients experiencing DKA?

6. What additional blood level (other than blood glucose) is monitored in diabetic patients on a regular basis? What is its significance in treating diabetes? What results indicate (1) good control, (2) fair control, and (3) poor control of blood glucose levels?

7. What is an ADA diet?

Additional orders for T.C. include VS q 4 hr, glucose checks ac and at bedtime, CBC, BMP, Hgb A_{1c}, and urinalysis daily, falls precautions, I&O, daily weight, consult ophthalmology, diabetic educator, and social services.

Medication orders include:

· Glargine insulin 4 units subcut, q AM
· Magnesium hydroxide/aluminum hydroxide/simethicone suspension 30 mL PO q 4 hr PRN
· Acetaminophen 650 mg PO q 4-6 hr PRN
· sliding scale insulin coverage
   · Lispro insulin 2 units subcut if AC and bedtime BS 151-200
   · Lispro insulin 4 units subcut if AC and bedtime BS 201-250
   · Lispro insulin 6 units subcut if AC and bedtime BS 251-300
   · Lispro insulin 8 units subcut if AC and bedtime BS 301-350
   · Lispro insulin 10 units subcut if AC and bedtime BS 351-400
   · Lispro insulin 12 units subcut if AC and bedtime BS 401-450
   · Call PCP if AC and bedtime BS >451
· IV $D_5\frac{1}{2}$ NS at 150 mL/hr

8. What type of insulins are glargine and lispro? Provide the onset, peak, and duration of both.

INSULIN	ONSET	PEAK	DURATION
Glargine			
Lispro			

9. What type of insulin is given IV to patients in DKA? What are its onset, peak, and duration?

10. What is the purpose of T.C. receiving 150 mL/hr of $D_5\frac{1}{2}$ NS in addition to her taking oral fluids and food?

ASSESSMENT UPDATE

1130 VS T 37° C (98.6°F), BP 120/62, P 72 and regular, R 18 and unlabored. O_2 sat 99% on RA. Bilateral leg pain at 4/10 accompanied by numbness and tingling. Urinalysis normal.

$$\begin{array}{c|c|c}
140 & 104 & 18 \\
\hline
3.2 & 27 & 1.0
\end{array} \bigg\rangle 180$$

$$9.7 \bigg\rangle \begin{array}{c} 11.6 \\ \hline 36 \end{array} \bigg\langle 243$$

Hgb A_{1c} 11%

11. Describe diabetic neuropathy, retinopathy, and paresthesia, and how they affect individuals with diabetes.

12. At noon, your UAP reports that T.C.'s blood sugar is 256, which means that she needs insulin coverage. What type of insulin will you give her, and how many units will you administer? What action do you need to take, in addition to the three checks and six rights of medication administration, before giving T.C. her coverage?

13. In what time period should you assess T.C. most closely for a potential hypoglycemic response following administration of her insulin coverage?

14. When you go in to T.C.'s room to check on her at 1300, you notice that she has not eaten more than 20% of her lunch, and she is pale, diaphoretic, and acting nervous. What action should you take?

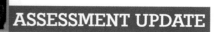

ASSESSMENT UPDATE

1305 VS T 36.8°C (98.2°F), BP 142/74, P 102 and regular, R 22 and shallow. O₂ sat 97% on RA. BS 53.

15. In light of the 1305 assessment findings, what nursing interventions should you initiate? Explain the procedure for treating patients with blood glucose levels <70.

16. In light of T.C.'s unstable blood glucose levels her PCP discontinues her glargine insulin and changes her programmed insulin order to NPH insulin 30 units and regular insulin 10 units subcut q AM. What type of insulin are NPH and regular? Provide the onset, peak, and duration of both.

INSULIN	ONSET	PEAK	DURATION
NPH			
Regular			

17. The next morning you are assigned to take care of T.C. again. In preparation for administering her new programmed insulin orders, describe the step-by-step procedure for mixing insulin.

18. Explain the role of the ophthalmologist, diabetic educator, and social worker in T.C.'s care. Identify two additional members of the health care team that may be important to consult.

19. Complete the CCM at the end of this case study or online in the CCM Creator on Evolve. Be sure to include all of the assessment data, medications (including changes), and lab results before developing a patient centered plan of care for T.C. with three nursing diagnoses pertinent to her current condition while hospitalized.

Conceptual Care Map

Medications

IV Sites/Fluids/Rate

Past Medical/Surgical History

Student Name_____

Patient Initials _____ Room # _____ Admission Date _____

Code Status _____ Today's Date _____ Age_____ Gender _____

Weight _____ Height _____ Braden Score _____

Diet _____ Activity _____

Religion _____ Allergies _____

Admitting Diagnoses/Chief Complaint

Assessment Data

Lab Values/Diagnostic Test Results

BMP

CBC

Misc Lab Values/Diagnostic Test Results

Treatments

Primary Nursing Diagnosis	Nursing Diagnosis 2	Nursing Diagnosis 3
Supporting Data	Supporting Data	Supporting Data
STG/NOC	STG/NOC	STG/NOC
Interventions/NIC with Rationale	Interventions/NIC with Rationale	Interventions/NIC with Rationale
Rationale Citation/EBP	Rationale Citation/EBP	Rationale Citation/EBP
Evaluation	Evaluation	Evaluation

ⓔ An interactive version of the Conceptual Care Map is on Evolve.

CASE STUDY

29

Erika Pratt

Name/s _____ Date _____

Patient Assignment

E.P. is a 48-year-old married mother of two diagnosed with breast cancer 5 months ago. She is a direct admit from her oncologist's office with complaints of mouth sores, extreme fatigue, and weakness. Her mouth sores have made it too painful to eat, and she has not been out of bed except to go to the bathroom for 2 days. Her husband of 25 years is with her. They have twins, both of whom are in college out of state.

E.P. had a left mastectomy with reconstruction for breast CA 4 months ago and began chemotherapy 1 month later. She returned to work part time as an English professor 2 weeks after her first round of chemo treatments. Ten days ago, she received her third chemotherapy treatment. E.P.'s admitting diagnosis is R/O neutropenia.

Initial Assessment

1030 VS T 37.5° C (99.5° F), BP 112/52, P 98 and regular, R 24 and shallow. O_2 sat 96% on RA. Pain 2/10 in both legs described as aching and intermittent. Pain of 6/10 in mouth secondary to multiple inflamed areas on her tongue, gums, and hard palate. A&O×4. Lungs diminished in lower lobes, clear upper lobes bilaterally. SOB while walking to the bathroom. Apical pulse 98 bpm. Abdomen is soft, flat with BS×4. No N&V. MAE. Denies difficulty with urinating or bowel elimination. Capillary refill <3, pedal pulses 2+ bilaterally, slight edema and redness noted in R calf. E.P. weighs 47 kg (104 lb) and is 167.6 cm (66 in) tall. She is a full code with advance directives in place. Braden score is 21.

1. What is neutropenia? List a minimum of four clinical manifestations of neutropenia.

2. When is neutropenia most likely to occur in patients undergoing chemotherapy?

3. What is the primary concern associated with neutropenia?

4. As the charge nurse who will be admitting E.P. today, identify the type of room to which you will assign her.

Admission Orders

Admit to unit in protective isolation. VS q 8 hr. No BP or blood draws in left arm. Up ad lib. Falls precautions. Daily weight. Neutropenic diet with supplements. Use soft mouth swabs for oral care. Strict I&O. CBC with ANC and BMP daily, and prealbumin today. Initiate IV $D_5W/0.9NS$ @ 100 mL/hr. Start Ciprofloxacin 500 mg IVPB q 12 hr. May have acetaminophen 650 mg PO q 4-6 hr PRN. Ultrasound R calf. Orthostatic BP check. Consider initiating short-term total parenteral nutrition (TPN) in consultation with patient in the AM.

5. Describe protective isolation including its purpose, and provide key guidelines with rationales for maintaining this type of isolation.

6. Briefly explain the rationale for not taking any blood pressure (BP) readings or blood draws from E.P.'s left arm.

7. What is the rationale for doing orthostatic BP checks on E.P.?

8. E.P. has significant oral mucositis. Provide a brief explanation of its etiology.

9. Although there is varied support for neutropenic dietary restrictions in research at present, most neutropenic patients are encouraged to maintain at least a modified neutropenic diet to prevent exposure to pathogens while they are most susceptible to infection. List guidelines for a neutropenic diet that can be used in patient education. Provide an online link to which a patient can be referred to for support.

10. Provide a rationale for assessing E.P.'s weight on a daily basis and maintaining her strict I&O order.

11. What is total parenteral nutrition (TPN)? What is its purpose?

12. What is the most critical lab value to monitor for a patient who is admitted with the diagnosis of R/O neutropenia? Provide a rationale for your answer.

13. Briefly describe the purpose of monitoring E.P.'s prealbumin blood level.

ASSESSMENT UPDATE

1842 E.P. consumed less than 10% of her dinner and drank only 250 mL of water with her meal. She explains that it hurts to swallow or put anything in her mouth. She is complaining of more pain (3/10), which has increased in constancy, in her R calf. She is on call for her ultrasound. E.P.'s husband went home to feed the family dog and call their twins to notify them of their mother's hospitalization. Lab results are as follows:

CBC
WBC 3×10^9/L
Hgb 11
Hct 32%
Plt 185×10^9/L

ANC 650/mm^3

Blood cultures—pending

BMP
Na 138 mEq/L
K^+ 4.2 mEq/L
Cl 104 mmol/L
CO_2 26 mmol/L
BUN 18 mg/dL
Creat 0.9 mg/dL
Glucose 72 mg/dL

Prealbumin 12 mg/dL

14. There is a new graduate nurse orienting on your unit. He asks you if you need to be taking chemotherapy precautions when caring for E.P. Explain what hospital-based chemotherapy precautions involve and when they are necessary while caring for patients undergoing chemotherapy treatments.

15. Develop a care plan for E.P. by recording all of E.P.'s assessment data, medication orders, and treatment orders in the CCM. Be sure to include all required medication information and lab result analysis, including the normal range and an explanation for each abnormal lab value, when completing your plan of care.

ASSESSMENT UPDATE

2021 E.P.'s call light is activated. When you enter her room, E.P. is sitting in a chair several feet from her bed. She complains of a sudden onset of severe chest pain, and she appears diaphoretic and extremely short of breath.

16. What is the most likely etiology of E.P.'s sudden change in physical condition? Give a brief explanation of the etiology.

17. Identify a minimum of five nursing interventions that you need to initiate immediately upon entering E.P.'s room and observing her condition.

18. E.P. is transferred to the medical intensive care unit (MICU). Provide a brief explanation of nursing actions you need to take related to her transfer.

Conceptual Care Map

Medications

IV Sites/Fluids/Rate

Past Medical/Surgical History

Student Name _____

Patient Initials _____ Room # _____ Admission Date _____

CODE Status _____ Today's Date _____ Age_____ Gender _____

Weight _____ Height _____ Braden Score _____

Diet _____ Activity _____

Religion _____ Allergies _____

Admitting Diagnoses/Chief Complaint

Assessment Data

Lab Values/Diagnostic Test Results

BMP

CBC

Misc Lab Values/Diagnostic Test Results

Treatments

Primary Nursing Diagnosis	Nursing Diagnosis 2	Nursing Diagnosis 3
Supporting Data	Supporting Data	Supporting Data
STG/NOC	STG/NOC	STG/NOC
Interventions/NIC with Rationale	Interventions/NIC with Rationale	Interventions/NIC with Rationale
Rationale Citation/EBP	Rationale Citation/EBP	Rationale Citation/EBP
Evaluation	Evaluation	Evaluation

ⓔ An interactive version of the Conceptual Care Map is on Evolve.

Name/s _____   **Date** _____

Patient Assignment

K.V. is a 72-year-old male who was brought to the emergency department (ED) by the emergency medical technician (EMT) squad. He collapsed at home, and his wife called 911. Assessment by the squad revealed a BP of 94/58, P 104 and regular, R 22 and slightly labored, O_2 saturation 92% on RA. T 38.6° C (101.5° F). His wife stated that he did not feel well that morning and was having difficulty urinating. The EMTs started an IV of 0.9% NS at 200 mL/hr, placed him on 2 L O_2 via nasal cannula, and transported him to the ED.

Initial Assessment

1105 VS: T 38.9° C (102° F), BP 88/50, P 110 and regular, R 24 and slightly labored. O_2 saturation 94% on 2 L O_2 via nasal cannula. Denies pain. A&O to person but confused about time, place, and situation. PER-RLA. Lungs clear. Apical pulse is 112 and regular. BS present in all four quadrants. Abdomen is soft and nontender. Skin very warm, flushed, and dry. Capillary refill >3 seconds. MAE. Pedal pulses 3+ bilaterally. Slight edema in lower extremities. IV infusing into right forearm through a 22-gauge catheter. No redness or swelling at site. Height 177.8 cm (70 in). Weight 84 kg (184.8 lb). BMI 26.5.

During your assessment, K.V.'s wife states that he had an UTI and prostatitis once before, about 3 years ago. At that time, he had burning upon urination and had difficulty emptying his bladder. He went to urgent care and was prescribed an oral antibiotic. She states that "he never got this sick." They had been debating this morning about calling his doctor or going to urgent care when he began feeling "light-headed" and then collapsed. He does not take any regular medications and has no chronic medical problems.

1. What concerns do you have about K.V. after your initial assessment?

2. You suspect that K.V. is exhibiting signs of sepsis and that his condition is urgent since you know that sepsis can lead to severe sepsis and septic shock. What assessment findings made you suspect sepsis? What should you do next?

3. What is sepsis? How can sepsis lead to septic shock?

ASSESSMENT UPDATE

The ED team is immediately alerted about K.V.'s abnormal vital signs. Blood and urine cultures are ordered. Other orders include insert Foley catheter; increase IV rate of 0.9% NS to 1000 mL/hr × 1 hr then 200 mL/hr pending lab results; CBC, BMP, and lactate level; chest x-ray; cardiac monitoring; O_2 at 2 L/min via nasal cannula; levofloxacin 750 mg IV infusion daily, start as soon as blood and urine cultures are obtained.

You increase the IV rate to 1000 mL/hr at 1120 and start another IV access line with a 22-gauge catheter in the left hand. Another ED nurse inserts the Foley catheter and meets resistance. He asks the patient to cough and is able to insert the catheter past the resistance. 250 mL of cloudy, amber urine flow out through the catheter immediately. The nurse clamps the tubing for 10 minutes and then obtains the urine culture specimen through the specimen port. The lab technician draws the blood work including cultures. The pharmacy sends the levofloxacin premixed in a 150 mL bag of D5W. The instructions read: infuse over 90 minutes.

4. Given K.V.'s age, history of difficulty urinating and previous prostatitis and UTI, and the fact that the nurse met resistance when inserting the catheter, what are the two most likely sources of infection?

5. What are the four interventions that are recommended by the Society of Critical Care Medicine for sepsis patients within the first 3 hours of treatment?

6. Mean arterial pressure (MAP) can be calculated in mm Hg noninvasively using the formula:

$$\frac{\text{Systolic BP (SBP)} + 2 \; (\text{Diastolic BP [DBP]})}{3} = \text{MAP in mm Hg}$$

The goal of sepsis treatment is to keep the MAP ≥65. Calculate K.V.'s MAP when he arrived at the ED.

7. What are the next three interventions that are to be completed within the first 6 hours of treatment recommended by the Society of Critical Care Medicine?

8. What is the purpose of obtaining a lactate level?

9. If K.V.'s lactate level is above 4 mmol/L, how much fluid should he receive within the first 3 hours of treatment?

10. What is the classification of levofloxacin? What is the rationale behind waiting to start the IV levofloxacin until the cultures are obtained?

11. At what rate will you run the levofloxacin on the IV infusion pump through the left hand access site?

1215 VS: T 38.6° C (101.5° F), BP 94/56, P 104 and regular, R 22. O_2 saturation 96% on 2 L O_2 via nasal can-nula. Denies pain. Apical pulse is 106 and regular. The 1000 mL of IV is almost finished infusing. Alert but confused. Wife at bedside. Braden score 21. NKDA.

Lab Results: *CBC: Hgb 15 g/dL, Hct 48%, WBC 15,000/mm^3, Platelets 500 × 10^9/L.*

BMP: sodium 142 mEq/L, K 4.8 mEq/L, chloride 102 mEq/L, bicarb 19 mEq/L, BUN 20 mg/dL, creatinine 1.8 mg/dL, glucose 140 mg/dL;

Lactate level: 4.1 mmol/L (0.6-2.2).

Urine and blood cultures pending.

Chest x-ray: normal

New orders: *1500 mL 0.9% NS IV, infuse over 2 hours, then IV of 0.9% NS infuse at 100 mL/hr. Transfer to ICU. Repeat CBC, BMP, and lactate level at 1400. Bed rest. Clear liquid diet. Monitor I&O and daily weights. Full code.*

12. Insert K.V.'s lab values into the CCM. Interpret the lab values on the CCM.

13. 1000 mL of the 1500 mL of 0.9% NS IV fluids has infused. You hang the bag of 500 mL of 0.9% NS at 1340 and set the pump at 750 mL/hr. The first dose of levofloxacin has infused. You prepare K.V. for transfer to the ICU. What will be important to include in your report to the ICU nurse?

14. As the ICU nurse, list in order of priority at least six nursing diagnoses or patient problems for K.V.

15. Complete a CCM for Case Study 30 in this book or in the CCM Creator on Evolve for K.V. Use the top three nursing diagnoses or patient problems from the previous question, and formulate a plan of care for him. Include all data from the ED and his course of treatment so far. Use the Assessment Update at 1500 to evaluate the plan of care.

ASSESSMENT UPDATE

1500 VS: T 38.2° C (100.8° F), BP 98/60, P 100 and regular, R 22. O_2 saturation 98% on 2 L O_2 via nasal cannula. Denies pain. A&O×4. PERRLA. Lungs clear. Apical pulse is 100 and regular. BS present in all four quadrants. Abdomen is soft and nontender. Skin warm and dry. Capillary refill <2 seconds. MAE. Pedal pulses 2+ bilaterally. Slight edema in lower extremities. IV infusing into right forearm through a 22-gauge catheter. Saline lock in left hand, 22 gauge. No redness or swelling at sites. I&O totals for shift 1100-1500: intake 2800 mL; output 800 mL.

K.V.'s wife is in the ICU waiting room contacting their children to give them an update of their father's condition. She asks her son to come to the hospital to be with her. She states that K.V. "had prostatitis in the past but didn't get this sick." She says that "she didn't realize how sick he was until he collapsed." She states that his pastor from their Presbyterian church wanted to come to the hospital, but she asked him to wait until tomorrow.

1400 lab results: CBC: normal except WBC 14,500/mm³, platelets 480 x 10⁹/L
BMP: normal except creatinine 1.5 mg/dL, glucose 126 mg/dL
Lactate level: 3.8 mmol/L (0.6-2.2)

16. What positive changes have occurred in K.V.'s assessment since he arrived at the ED? Include a calculation of his current MAP.

17. How have his lab results changed? Give rationales.

18. What interventions for K.V. are important for the ICU nurse to initiate during the next several hours? What interventions are important for his family?

Conceptual Care Map

Medications

IV Sites/Fluids/Rate

Past Medical/Surgical History

Student Name_____

Patient Initials _____ Room # _____ Admission Date _____

CODE Status _____ Today's Date _____ Age_____ Gender _____

Weight _____ Height _____ Braden Score _____

Diet _____ Activity _____

Religion _____ Allergies _____

Admitting Diagnoses/Chief Complaint

Assessment Data

Lab Values/Diagnostic Test Results

BMP

CBC

Misc Lab Values/Diagnostic Test Results

Treatments

Primary Nursing Diagnosis	Nursing Diagnosis 2	Nursing Diagnosis 3
Supporting Data	Supporting Data	Supporting Data
STG/NOC	STG/NOC	STG/NOC
Interventions/NIC with Rationale	Interventions/NIC with Rationale	Interventions/NIC with Rationale
Rationale Citation/EBP	Rationale Citation/EBP	Rationale Citation/EBP
Evaluation	Evaluation	Evaluation

e An interactive version of the Conceptual Care Map is on Evolve.

Illustration Credits

Chapter 1

Fig. 1.14, From Bulechek G, Butcher H, Dochterman J, et al. *Nursing interventions classification [NIC].* 6th ed. St. Louis: Elsevier; 2013 and Moorhead S, Johnson M, Mass M, et al. *Nursing outcomes classification [NOC].* 5th ed. St. Louis: Elsevier; 2013.

Chapter 2

Fig. 2.1, © istock.com

Fig. 2.2, © istock.com

Fig. 2.4, © istock.com

Chapter 3

Fig. 3.1, © istock.com

Fig. 3.2, © istock.com

Chapter 4

Fig. 4.1, © istock.com

Fig. 4.2, © istock.com

Fig. 4.3, © istock.com

Chapter 5

Fig. 5.3, © Shutterstock.com

Fig. 5.4, Copyright 2015 by R. Alfaro-LeFevre. http://www.alfaroteachsmart.co/

Fig. 5.5, © istock.com

Fig. 5.6, From Bob Christy, Kent State University, Kent, Ohio.

Case Study 1, 2, 3, 4, 5, 6, 7, 8, 9, 10, 11, 12, 13, 14, 15, 16, 17, 18, 19, 20, 21, 22, 23, 24, 25, 26, 27, 28, 29, 30

Case Study figure © istock.com

Case Study 7, Question 9

Used with permission of the National Pressure Ulcer Advisory Panel, © NPUAP.

Case Study 20, Question 9

From Lewis SL, Bucher L, Heitkemper MM, et al. *Medical-surgical nursing: assessment and management of clinical problems.* 10th ed. St. Louis: Elsevier; 2017.

Case Study 23, Question 6

Photos from Elsevier: *Clinical skills: Essentials collection,* St. Louis: Elsevier; 2017.

Line drawing from deWit SC, O'Neill P. *Fundamental concepts and skills for nursing.* 4th ed. St. Louis: Elsevier; 2014.

Case Study 26, Question 8

From Walker BR, Colledge NR, Ralston SH, et al. *Davidson's principles and practice of medicine.* 21st ed. London: Elsevier; 2010.

APPENDIX A

NANDA Definitions from Nursing Diagnoses: Definitions and Classification 2015–2017, ed 10

Activity intolerance Insufficient physiological or psychological energy to endure or complete required or desired daily activities.

Acute confusion Abrupt onset of reversible disturbances of consciousness, attention, cognition, and perception that develop over a short period of time.

Acute pain An unpleasant sensory and emotional experience associated with actual or potential tissue damage, or described in terms of such damage (International Association for the Study of Pain); sudden or slow onset of any intensity from mild to severe with an anticipated or predictable end.

Anxiety Vague, uneasy feeling of discomfort or dread accompanied by an autonomic response (the source is often nonspecific or unknown to the individual); a feeling of apprehension caused by anticipation of danger. It is an alerting sign that warns of impending danger and enables the individual to take measures to deal with threat.

Autonomic dysreflexia Life-threatening, uninhibited sympathetic response of the nervous system to a noxious stimulus after a spinal cord injury at T7 or above.

Bathing self-care deficit Impaired ability to perform or complete bathing activities for self.

Bowel incontinence Change in normal bowel habits characterized by involuntary passage of stool.

Caregiver role strain Difficulty in performing family/significant other caregiver role.

Chronicconfusion Irreversible, long-standing, and/or progressive deterioration of intellect and personality characterized by decreased ability to interpret environmental stimuli

and decreased capacity for intellectual thought processes, and manifested by disturbances of memory, orientation, and behavior.

Chronic functional constipation Infrequent or difficult evacuation of feces, which has been present for at least three of the prior 12 months.

Chronic low self-esteem Longstanding negative self-evaluating/feelings about self or self-capabilities.

Chronic pain syndrome Recurrent or persistent pain that has lasted at least 3 months and that significantly affects daily functioning or well-being.

Chronic pain Unpleasant sensory and emotional experience associated with actual or potential tissue damage, or described in terms of such damage (International Association for the Study of Pain); sudden or slow onset of any intensity from mild to severe, constant or recurring without an anticipated or predictable end and a duration of greater than 3 months.

Chronic sorrow Cyclical, recurring, and potentially progressive pattern of pervasive sadness experienced (by a parent, caregiver, individual with chronic illness or disability) in response to continual loss throughout the trajectory of an illness or disability.

Complicated grieving A disorder that occurs after the death of a significant other, in which the experience of distress accompanying bereavement fails to follow normative expectations and manifests in functional impairment.

Compromised family coping A usually supportive primary person (family member, significant other, or close friend) provides insufficient, ineffective, or compromised support, comfort, assistance, or encouragement that may be needed by the client to manage or master adaptive tasks related to his or her health challenge.

Constipation Decrease in normal frequency of defecation accompanied by difficult or incomplete passage of stool and/or passage of excessively hard, dry stool.

Contamination Exposure to environmental contaminants in doses sufficient to cause adverse health effects.

Death anxiety Vague, uneasy feeling of discomfort or dread generated by perceptions of a real or imagined threat to one's existence.

Decisional conflict Uncertainty about course of action to be taken when choice among competing actions involves risk, loss, or challenge to values and beliefs.

Decreased cardiac output Inadequate blood pumped by the heart to meet the metabolic demands of the body.

Decreased intracranial adaptive capacity Intracranial fluid dynamic mechanisms that normally compensate for increases in intracranial volumes are compromised, resulting in repeated disproportionate increases in intracranial pressure (ICP) in response to a variety of noxious and non-noxious stimuli.

Defensive coping Repeated projection of falsely positive self-evaluation based on a self-protective pattern that defends against underlying perceived threats to positive self-regard.

Deficient community health Presence of one or more health problems or factors that deter wellness or increase the risk of health problems experienced by an aggregate.

Deficient diversional activity Decreased stimulation from (or interest or engagement in) recreational or leisure activities.

Deficient fluid volume Decreased intravascular, interstitial, and/or intracellular fluid. This refers to dehydration, water loss alone without change in sodium level.

Deficient knowledge Absence or deficiency of cognitive information related to a specific topic.

Delayed surgical recovery Extension of the number of postoperative days required to initiate and perform activities that maintain life, health, and well-being.

Diarrhea Passage of loose, unformed stools.

Disabled family coping Behavior of primary person (family member, significant other, or close friend) that disables his or her capacities and the client's capacities to effectively address tasks essential to either person's adaptation to the health challenge.

Disorganized infant behavior Disintegrated physiological and neurobehavioral responses of infant to the environment.

Disturbed body image Confusion in mental picture of one's physical self.

Disturbed personal identity Inability to maintain an integrated and complete perception of self.

Disturbed sleep pattern Time-limited interruptions of sleep amount and quality due to external factors.

Dressing self-care deficit Impaired ability to perform or complete dressing activities for self.

Dysfunctional family processes Psychosocial, spiritual, and physiological functions of the family unit are chronically disorganized, which leads to conflict, denial of problems, resistance to change, ineffective problem-solving, and a series of self-perpetuating crises.

Dysfunctional gastrointestinal motility Increased, decreased, ineffective, or lack of peristaltic activity within the gastrointestinal system.

Dysfunctional ventilatory weaning response Inability to adjust to lowered levels of mechanical ventilator support that interrupts and prolongs the weaning process.

Excess fluid volume Increased isotonic fluid retention.

Fatigue An overwhelming, sustained sense of exhaustion and decreased capacity for physical and mental work at the usual level.

Fear Response to perceived threat that is consciously recognized as a danger.

Feeding self-care deficit Impaired ability to perform or complete self-feeding activities.

Frail elderly syndrome Dynamic state of unstable equilibrium that affects the older individual experiencing deterioration in one or more domain of health (physical, functional, psychological, or social) and leads to increased susceptibility to adverse health effects, particularly disability.

Functional urinary incontinence Inability of a usually continent person to reach the toilet in time to avoid unintentional loss of urine.

Grieving A normal complex process that includes emotional, physical, spiritual, social, and intellectual responses and behaviors by which individuals, families, and communities incorporate an actual, anticipated, or perceived loss into their daily lives.

Hopelessness Subjective state in which an individual sees limited or no alternatives or personal choices available and is unable to mobilize energy on own behalf.

Hyperthermia Core body temperature above the normal diurnal range due to failure of thermoregulation.

Hypothermia Core body temperature below normal diurnal range due to failure of thermoregulation.

Imbalanced nutrition: less than body requirements Intake of nutrients insufficient to meet metabolic needs.

Impaired bed mobility Limitation of independent movement from one bed position to another.

Impaired comfort Perceived lack of ease, relief, and transcendence in physical, psychospiritual, environmental, cultural, and/or social dimensions.

Impaired dentition Disruption in tooth development/ eruption patterns or structural integrity of individual teeth.

Impaired emancipated decision-making A process of choosing a health care decision that does not include personal knowledge and/or consideration of social norms, or does not occur in a flexible environment, resulting in decisional dissatisfaction.

Impaired gas exchange Excess or deficit in oxygenation and/or carbon dioxide elimination at the alveolar-capillary membrane.

Impaired home maintenance Inability to independently maintain a safe growth-promoting immediate environment.

Impaired memory Inability to remember or recall bits of information or behavioral skills.

Impaired mood regulation A mental state characterized by shifts in mood or affect and which is comprised of a constellation of affective, cognitive, somatic, and/or physiological manifestations varying from mild to severe.

Impaired oral mucous membrane Injury to the lips, soft tissue, buccal cavity, and/or oropharynx.

Impaired parenting Inability of the primary caretaker to create, maintain, or regain an environment that promotes the optimum growth and development of the child.

Impaired physical mobility Limitation in independent, purposeful physical movement of the body or of one or more extremities.

Impaired religiosity Impaired ability to exercise reliance on beliefs and/or participate in rituals of a particular faith tradition.

Impaired resilience Decreased ability to sustain a pattern of positive responses to an adverse situation or crisis.

Impaired sitting Limitation of ability to independently and purposefully attain and/or maintain a rest position that is supported by the buttocks and thighs, in which the torso is upright.

Impaired skin integrity Altered epidermis and/or dermis.

Impaired social interaction Insufficient or excessive quantity or ineffective quality of social exchange.

Impaired spontaneous ventilation Decreased energy reserves resulting in an inability to maintain independent breathing that is adequate to support life.

Impaired standing Limitation of ability to independently and purposefully attain and/or maintain the body in an upright position from feet to head.

Impaired swallowing Abnormal functioning of the swallowing mechanism associated with deficits in oral, pharyngeal, or esophageal structure or function.

Impaired tissue integrity Damage to the mucous membrane, cornea, integumentary system, muscular fascia, muscle, tendon, bone, cartilage, joint capsule, and/or ligament.

Impaired transfer ability Limitation of independent movement between two nearby surfaces.

Impaired urinary elimination Dysfunction in urine elimination.

Impaired verbal communication Decreased, delayed, or absent ability to receive, process, transmit, and/or use a system of symbols.

Impaired walking Limitation of independent movement within the environment on foot.

Impaired wheelchair mobility Limitation of independent operation of wheelchair within environment.

Ineffective activity planning Inability to prepare for a set of actions fixed in time and under certain conditions.

Ineffective airway clearance Inability to clear secretions or obstructions from the respiratory tract to maintain a clear airway.

Ineffective breastfeeding Difficulty providing milk to an infant or young child directly from the breasts, which may compromise nutritional status of the infant/child.

Ineffective breathing pattern Inspiration and/or expiration that does not provide adequate ventilation.

Ineffective childbearing process Pregnancy and childbirth process and care of the newborn that does not match the environmental context, norms, and expectation.

Ineffective community coping A pattern of community activities for adaptation and problem solving that is unsatisfactory for meeting the demands or needs of the community.

Ineffective coping Inability to form a valid appraisal of the stressors, inadequate choices of practiced responses, and/or inability to use available resources.

Ineffective denial Conscious or unconscious attempt to disavow the knowledge or meaning of an event to reduce anxiety and/or fear, leading to the detriment of health.

Ineffective family health management A pattern of regulating and integrating into family processes a program for the treatment of illness and its sequelae that is unsatisfactory for meeting specific health goals.

Ineffective health maintenance Inability to identify, manage, and/or seek out help to maintain health.

Ineffective health management Pattern of regulating and integrating into daily living a therapeutic regimen for the treatment of illness and its sequelae that is unsatisfactory for meeting specific health goals.

Ineffective impulse control A pattern of performing rapid, unplanned reactions to internal or external stimuli without regard for the negative consequences of these reactions to the impulsive individual or to others.

Ineffective infant feeding pattern Impaired ability of an infant to suck or coordinate the suck/swallow response resulting in inadequate oral nutrition for metabolic needs.

Ineffective peripheral tissue perfusion Decrease in blood circulation to the periphery that may compromise health.

Ineffective protection Decrease in the ability to guard self from internal or external threats such as illness or injury.

Ineffective relationship A pattern of mutual partnership that is insufficient to provide for each other's needs.

Ineffective role performance A pattern of behavior and self-expression that does not match the environmental context, norms, and expectations.

Ineffective sexuality pattern Expressions of concern regarding own sexuality.

Ineffective thermoregulation Temperature fluctuation between hypothermia and hyperthermia.

Insomnia A disruption in amount and quality of sleep that impairs functioning.

Insufficient breast milk Low production of maternal breast milk.

Interrupted breastfeeding Break in the continuity of providing milk to an infant or young child directly from the breasts, which may compromise breastfeeding success and/or nutritional status of the infant/child.

Interrupted family processes Change in family relationships and/or functioning.

Labile emotional control Uncontrollable outbursts of exaggerated and involuntary emotional expression.

Labor pain Sensory and emotional experience that varies from pleasant to unpleasant, associated with labor and childbirth.

Latex allergy response A hypersensitive reaction to natural latex rubber products.

Moral distress Response to the inability to carry out one's chosen ethical/moral decision/action.

Nausea A subjective phenomenon of an unpleasant feeling in the back of the throat and stomach, which may or may not result in vomiting.

Neonatal jaundice The yellow-orange tint of the neonate's skin and mucous membranes that occurs after 24 hours of life as a result of unconjugated bilirubin in the circulation.

Noncompliance Behavior of person and/or caregiver that fails to coincide with a health-promoting or therapeutic plan agreed on by the person (and/or family and/or community) and health care professional. In the presence of an agreed-on, health-promoting, or therapeutic plan, person's or caregiver's behavior is fully or partly nonadherent and may lead to clinically ineffective or partially effective outcomes.

Obesity A condition in which an individual accumulates abnormal or excessive fat for age and gender that exceeds overweight.

Overflow urinary incontinence Involuntary loss of urine associated with overdistention of the bladder.

Overweight A condition in which an individual accumulates abnormal or excessive fat for age and gender.

Parental role conflict Parental experience of role confusion and conflict in response to crisis.

Perceived constipation Self-diagnosis of constipation combined with abuse of laxatives, enemas, and/or suppositories to ensure a daily bowel movement.

Post-trauma syndrome Sustained maladaptive response to a traumatic, overwhelming event.

Powerlessness The lived experience of lack of control over a situation, including a perception that one's actions do not significantly affect an outcome.

Rape-trauma syndrome Sustained maladaptive response to a forced, violent, sexual penetration against the victim's will and consent.

Readiness for enhanced breastfeeding A pattern of providing milk to an infant or young child directly from the breasts, which may be strengthened.

Readiness for enhanced childbearing process A pattern of preparing for and maintaining a healthy pregnancy, childbirth process, and care of the newborn for ensuring well-being, which can be strengthened.

Readiness for enhanced comfort A pattern of ease, relief, and transcendence in physical, psychospiritual, environmental, and/or social dimensions, which can be strengthened.

Readiness for enhanced communication A pattern of exchanging information and ideas with others, which can be strengthened.

Readiness for enhanced community coping A pattern of community activities for adaptation and problem-solving for meeting the demands or needs of the community, which can be strengthened.

Readiness for enhanced coping A pattern of cognitive and behavioral efforts to manage demands related to well-being, which can be strengthened.

Readiness for enhanced decision-making A pattern of choosing a course of action for meeting short- and long-term health-related goals, which can be strengthened.

Readiness for enhanced emancipated decision-making A process of choosing a healthcare decision that includes personal knowledge and/or consideration of social norms, which can be strengthened.

Readiness for enhanced family coping A pattern of management of adaptive tasks by primary person (family member, significant other, or close friend) involved with the client's health change, which can be strengthened.

Readiness for enhanced family processes A pattern of family functioning to support the well-being of family members, which can be strengthened.

Readiness for enhanced fluid balance A pattern of equilibrium between the fluid volume and chemical composition of body fluids, which can be strengthened.

Readiness for enhanced health management A pattern of regulating and integrating into daily living a therapeutic regimen for treatment of illness and its sequelae, which can be strengthened.

Readiness for enhanced hope A pattern of expectations and desires for mobilizing energy on one's own behalf, which can be strengthened.

Readiness for enhanced knowledge A pattern of cognitive information related to a specific topic, or its acquisition, which can be strengthened.

Readiness for enhanced nutrition A pattern of nutrient intake, which can be strengthened.

Readiness for enhanced organized infant behavior A pattern of modulation of the physiological and behavioral systems of functioning (i.e., autonomic, motor, state-organization, self-regulatory, and attentional-interactional systems) in an infant, which can be strengthened.

Readiness for enhanced parenting A pattern of providing an environment for children or other dependent person(s) to nurture growth and development, which can be strengthened.

Readiness for enhanced power A pattern of participating knowingly in change for well-being, which can be strengthened.

Readiness for enhanced relationship A pattern of mutual partnership to provide for each other's needs, which can be strengthened.

Readiness for enhanced religiosity A pattern of reliance on religious beliefs and/or participation in rituals of a particular faith tradition, which can be strengthened.

Readiness for enhanced resilience A pattern of positive responses to an adverse situation or crisis, which can be strengthened.

Readiness for enhanced self-care A pattern of performing activities for oneself to meet health-related goals, which can be strengthened.

Readiness for enhanced self-concept A pattern of perceptions or ideas about the self, which can be strengthened.

Readiness for enhanced sleep A pattern of natural, periodic suspension of relative consciousness to provide rest and sustain a desired lifestyle, which can be strengthened.

Readiness for enhanced spiritual well-being A pattern of experiencing and integrating meaning and purpose in life through connectedness with self, others, art, music, literature, nature, and/or a power greater than oneself, which can be strengthened.

Readiness for enhanced urinary elimination A pattern of urinary functions for meeting eliminatory needs, which can be strengthened.

Reflex urinary incontinence Involuntary loss of urine at somewhat predictable intervals when a specific bladder volume is reached.

Relocation stress syndrome Physiological and/or psychosocial disturbance following transfer from one environment to another.

Risk for activity intolerance Vulnerable to insufficient physiological or psychological energy to endure or complete required or desired daily activities, which may compromise health.

Risk for acute confusion Vulnerable to reversible disturbances of consciousness, attention, cognition, and perception that develop over a short period of time, which may compromise health.

Risk for adverse reaction to iodinated contrast media Vulnerable to noxious or unintended reaction associated with the use of iodinated contrast media that can occur within 7 days after contrast agent injection, which may compromise health.

Risk for allergy response Vulnerable to exaggerated immune response or reaction to substances, which may compromise health.

Risk for aspiration Vulnerable to entry of gastrointestinal secretions, oropharyngeal secretions, solids, or fluids to the tracheobronchial passages, which may compromise health.

Risk for autonomic dysreflexia Vulnerable to life-threatening, uninhibited response of the sympathetic nervous system post-spinal shock, in an individual with spinal cord injury or lesion at T6 or above (has been demonstrated in patients with injuries at T7 and T8), which may compromise health.

Risk for bleeding Vulnerable to a decrease in blood volume, which may compromise health.

Risk for caregiver role strain Vulnerable to difficulty in performing the family/significant other caregiver role, which may compromise health.

Risk for chronic functional constipation Vulnerable to infrequent or difficult evacuation of feces, which has been present nearly 3 of the prior 12 months, which may compromise health.

Risk for chronic low self-esteem Vulnerable to longstanding negative self-evaluating/feelings about self or self-capabilities, which may compromise health.

Risk for complicated grieving Vulnerable to a disorder that occurs after death of a significant other in which the experience of distress accompanying bereavement fails to follow normative expectations and manifests in functional impairment, which may compromise health.

Risk for compromised human dignity Vulnerable for perceived loss of respect and honor, which may compromise health.

Risk for constipation Vulnerable to a decrease in normal frequency of defecation accompanied by difficult or incomplete passage of stool, which may compromise health.

Risk for contamination Vulnerable to exposure to environmental contaminants, which may compromise health.

Risk for corneal injury Vulnerable to infection or inflammatory lesion in the corneal tissue that can affect superficial or deep layers, which may compromise health.

Risk for decreased cardiac output Vulnerable to inadequate blood pumped by the heart to meet metabolic demands of the body, which may compromise health.

Risk for decreased cardiac tissue perfusion Vulnerable to a decrease in cardiac (coronary) circulation, which may compromise health.

Risk for deficient fluid volume Vulnerable to experiencing decreased intravascular, interstitial, and/or intracellular fluid volumes, which may compromise health.

Risk for delayed development Vulnerable to delay of 25% or more in one or more of the areas of social or self-regulatory behavior, or in cognitive, language, gross, or fine motor skills, which may compromise health.

Risk for delayed surgical recovery Vulnerable to an extension of the number of postoperative days required to initiate and perform activities that maintain life, health, and well-being, which may compromise health.

Risk for disorganized infant behavior Vulnerable to alteration in integration and modulation of the physiological and behavioral systems of functioning (i.e., autonomic, motor, state-organization, self-regulatory, and attentional-interactional systems), which may compromise health.

Risk for disproportionate growth Vulnerable to growth above the 97th percentile or below the 3rd percentile for age, crossing two percentile channels, which may compromise health.

Risk for disturbed maternal–fetal dyad Vulnerable to disruption of the symbiotic maternal-fetal dyad as a result of comorbid or pregnancy-related conditions, which may compromise health.

Risk for disturbed personal identity Vulnerable to the inability to maintain an integrated and complete perception of self, which may compromise health.

Risk for disuse syndrome Vulnerable to deterioration of body systems as the result of prescribed or unavoidable musculoskeletal inactivity, which may compromise health.

Risk for dry eye Vulnerable to eye discomfort or damage to the cornea and conjunctiva due to reduced quantity or quality of tears to moisten the eye, which may compromise health.

Risk for dysfunctional gastrointestinal motility Vulnerable to a decrease in normal frequency of defecation accompanied by difficult or incomplete passage of stool, which may compromise health.

Risk for electrolyte imbalance Vulnerable to changes in serum electrolyte levels, which may compromise health.

Risk for falls Vulnerable to increased susceptibility to falling, which may cause physical harm and compromise health.

Risk for frail elderly syndrome Vulnerable to a dynamic state of unstable equilibrium that affects the older individual experiencing deterioration in one or more domains of health (physical, functional, or social) and leads to increased susceptibility to adverse health effects, in particular disability.

Risk for hypothermia Vulnerable to a failure of thermoregulation that may result in a core body temperature below the normal diurnal range, which may compromise health.

Risk for imbalanced body temperature Vulnerable to failure to maintain body temperature within normal parameters, which may compromise health.

Risk for imbalanced fluid volume Vulnerable to a decrease, increase, or rapid shift from one to the other of intravascular, interstitial, and/or intracellular fluid, which may compromise health. This refers to body fluid loss, gain, or both.

Risk for impaired attachment Vulnerable to disruption of the interactive process between parent/significant other and child that fosters the development of a protective and nurturing reciprocal relationship.

Risk for impaired cardiovascular function Vulnerable to internal or external causes that can damage one or more vital organs and the circulatory system itself.

Risk for impaired emancipated decision-making Vulnerable to a process of choosing a health care decision that does not include personal knowledge and/or considerations of social norms or does not occur in a flexible environment resulting in decisional satisfaction.

Risk for impaired liver function Vulnerable to a decrease in liver function, which may compromise health.

Risk for impaired oral mucous membrane Vulnerable to injury to the lips, soft tissues, buccal cavity, and/or oropharynx, which may compromise health.

Risk for impaired parenting Vulnerable to inability of the primary caretaker to create, maintain, or regain an environment that promotes the optimum growth and development of the child, which may compromise the well-being of the child.

Risk for impaired religiosity Vulnerable to an impaired ability to exercise reliance on religious beliefs and/or participate in rituals of a particular faith tradition, which may compromise health.

Risk for impaired resilience Vulnerable to decreased ability to sustain a pattern of positive response to an adverse situation or crisis, which may compromise health.

Risk for impaired skin integrity Vulnerable to alteration in epidermis and/or dermis, which may compromise health.

Risk for impaired tissue integrity Vulnerable to damage to the mucous membrane, cornea, integumentary system, muscular fascia, muscle, tendon, bone, cartilage, joint capsule, and/or ligament, which may compromise health.

Risk for ineffective activity planning Vulnerable to an inability to prepare for a set of actions fixed in time and under certain conditions, which may compromise health.

Risk for ineffective cerebral tissue perfusion Vulnerable to a decrease in cerebral tissue circulation, which may compromise health.

Risk for ineffective childbearing process Vulnerable to not matching environmental context, norms, and expectations of pregnancy, childbirth process, and the care of the newborn.

Risk for ineffective gastrointestinal perfusion Vulnerable to decrease in gastrointestinal circulation, which may compromise health.

Risk for ineffective peripheral tissue perfusion Vulnerable to a decrease in blood circulation to the periphery, which may compromise health.

Risk for ineffective relationship Vulnerable to developing a pattern that is insufficient for providing a mutual partnership to provide for each other's needs.

Risk for ineffective renal perfusion Vulnerable to a decrease in blood circulation to the kidney, which may compromise health.

Risk for infection Vulnerable to invasion and multiplication of pathogenic organisms, which may compromise health.

Risk for injury Vulnerable to physical damage due to environmental conditions interacting with the individual's adaptive and defensive resources, which may compromise health.

Risk for latex allergy response Vulnerable to a hypersensitive reaction to natural latex rubber products, which may compromise health.

Risk for loneliness Vulnerable to experiencing discomfort associated with a desire or need for more contact with others, which may compromise health.

Risk for neonatal jaundice Vulnerable to the yellow-orange tint of the neonate's skin and mucous membranes that occur after 24 hours of life as a result of unconjugated bilirubin in the circulation, which may compromise health.

Risk for other-directed violence Vulnerable to behaviors in which an individual demonstrates that he or she can be physically, emotionally, and/or sexually harmful to others.

Risk for overweight Vulnerable to abnormal or excessive fat accumulation for age and gender, which may compromise health.

Risk for perioperative hypothermia Vulnerable to an inadvertent drop in core body temperature below 36° C/96.8° F occurring one hour before to 24 hours after surgery, which may compromise health.

Risk for perioperative positioning injury Vulnerable to inadvertent anatomical and physical changes as a result of posture or equipment used during an invasive/surgical procedure, which may compromise health.

Risk for peripheral neurovascular dysfunction Vulnerable to disruption in the circulation, sensation, and motion of an extremity, which may compromise health.

Risk for poisoning Vulnerable to accidental exposure to, or ingestion of, drugs or dangerous products in sufficient doses, which may compromise health.

Risk for post-trauma syndrome Vulnerable to sustained maladaptive response to a traumatic, overwhelming event, which may compromise health.

Risk for powerlessness Vulnerable to the lived experience of lack of control over a situation, including a perception that one's actions do not significantly affect the outcome, which may compromise health.

Risk for pressure ulcer Vulnerable to localized injury to the skin and/or underlying tissue usually over a bony prominence as a result of pressure, or pressure in combination with shear (National Pressure Ulcer Advisory Panel [NPUAP], 2007). Updated Pressure Ulcer Stages available at: http://www.npuap.org/resources/educational-and-clinical-resources/npuap-pressure-injury-stages/.

Risk for relocation stress syndrome Vulnerable to physiological and/or psychosocial disturbance following transfer from one environment to another that may compromise health.

Risk for self-directed violence Vulnerable to behaviors in which an individual demonstrates that he or she can be physically, emotionally and/or sexually harmful to self.

Risk for self-mutilation Vulnerable to deliberate self-injurious behavior causing tissue damage with the intent of causing nonfatal injury to attain relief of tension.

Risk for shock Vulnerable to an inadequate blood flow to the body's tissues that may lead to life-threatening cellular dysfunction, which may compromise health.

Risk for situational low self-esteem Vulnerable to developing a negative perception of self-worth in response to a current situation, which may compromise health.

Risk for spiritual distress Vulnerable to an impaired ability to experience and integrate meaning and purpose in life through connectedness within self, literature, nature, and/or a power greater than oneself, which may compromise health.

Risk for sudden infant death syndrome Vulnerable to unpredicted death of an infant.

Risk for suffocation Vulnerable to inadequate air availability for inhalation, which may compromise health.

Risk for suicide Vulnerable to self-inflicted, life-threatening injury.

Risk for thermal injury Vulnerable to extreme temperature damage to skin and mucous membranes, which may compromise health.

Risk for trauma Vulnerable to accidental tissue injury (e.g., wound, burn, fracture), which may compromise health.

Risk for unstable blood glucose level Vulnerable to variation in blood glucose/sugar levels from the normal range, which may compromise health.

Risk for urge urinary incontinence Vulnerable to involuntary passage of urine occurring soon after a strong sensation or urgency to void, which may compromise health.

Risk for urinary tract injury Vulnerable to damage of the urinary tract structures from use of catheters, which may compromise health.

Risk for vascular trauma Vulnerable to damage to vein and its surrounding tissues related to the presence of a catheter and/or infusion solutions, which may compromise health.

Risk-prone health behavior Impaired ability to modify lifestyle/behaviors in a manner that improves health status.

Sedentary lifestyle Reports a habit of life that is characterized by a low physical activity level.

Self-mutilation Deliberate self-injurious behavior causing tissue damage with the intent of causing nonfatal injury to attain relief of tension.

Self-neglect A constellation of culturally framed behaviors involving one or more self-care activities in which there is a failure to maintain a socially accepted standard of health and well-being (Gibbons S, Lauder W, Luckwick R. (2006). Self-neglect: A proposed new NANDA diagnosis. *International Journal of Nursing Terminologies and Classification*. 2006;17(1):10-18).

Sexual dysfunction A state in which an individual experiences a change in sexual function during the sexual response phases of desire, excitation, and/or orgasm, which is viewed as unsatisfying, unrewarding, or inadequate.

Situational low self-esteem Development of a negative perception of self-worth in response to a current situation.

Sleep deprivation Prolonged periods of time without sleep (sustained natural, periodic suspension of relative consciousness).

Social isolation Aloneness experienced by the individual and perceived as imposed by others and as a negative or threatening state.

Spiritual distress A state of suffering related to the impaired ability to experience meaning in life through connections with self, others, world, or a superior being.

Stress overload Excessive amounts and types of demands that require action.

Stress urinary incontinence Sudden leakage of urine with activities that increase intra-abdominal pressure.

Toileting self-care deficit Impaired ability to perform or complete self-toileting activities.

Unilateral neglect Impairment in sensory and motor response, mental representation, and spatial attention of the body, and the corresponding environment, characterized by inattention to one side and overattention to the opposite side. Left-side neglect is more severe and persistent than right-side neglect.

Urge urinary incontinence Involuntary passage of urine occurring soon after a strong sense of urgency to void.

Urinary retention Incomplete emptying of the bladder.

Wandering Meandering, aimless or repetitive locomotion that exposes the individual to harm; frequently incongruent with boundaries, limits, or obstacles.

Herdman, T.H. and Kamitsuru, S. (Eds.): *Nursing Diagnoses - Definitions and Classification 2015-2017,* Copyright © 2017, 1994-2017 NANDA International. Used by arrangement with John Wiley & Sons, Inc.

APPENDIX B

Conceptual Care Map (CCM) Submission Checklist

Below are questions to ask yourself prior to submitting a conceptual care map for evaluation. Please take the time to read each section, and make sure your conceptual care map includes each aspect prior to turning in your conceptual care map to your faculty member.

General

Did you look at the CCM example entries throughout Chapter 1?	

Data Collection and Interpretation

Demographic Data

Are all of the demographic data recorded accurately?	
Date of care?	
Are all of the patient's medical diagnoses listed, including the admitting diagnosis/chief, complaint?	

Data Collection

Do your assessment data include data from every body system using a head-to-toe or body systems' organizational format?	
Did you remember to include any skin turgor findings, pedal pulses, and edema assessment?	
Are times listed indicating when key assessment data were collected (night shift report, head-to-toe assessment, time of intake and output collection, etc.)?	

Have you included the following data:	
Vital signs? Pain assessment (both before and after analgesic administration)?	
Are intake and output for the shift recorded?	
Color and quality of urine? Amount?	
Bowel movement frequency and consistency?	
Amount of diet taken?	
IV site assessment? (appearance, location, condition of dressing)	
Activities of daily living?	
Any subjective data (from the patient or family members)?	
Data regarding relevant spiritual, living, work, sexuality, or family dynamics?	

Medications

Are all of your patient's medications listed?	
Is the pharmacologic classification listed for each medication (i.e., loop diuretic, not just diuretic; opioid analgesic, not just analgesic)?	
Have you identified and listed the specific reason that you think your patient is receiving each medication?	

Lab Values/Diagnostic Test Results

Are all relevant labs listed and analyzed, including notation of normal versus ↑ or ↓?	
Is the normal reference range listed for all abnormal labs?	
Is the reason for any abnormalities listed for every abnormal lab related to your specific patient?	

Are at least all labs in the two lab skeletons included plus any others pertinent to your patient?	
Have you included other diagnostic test results that your patient has had x-rays, CT or MRI scans, scopes, etc.?	

Past Medical/Surgical History

Is your patient's past medical/surgical history included?	

Treatment

Are all treatments listed, including weight, intake and output, falls risk, deep vein thrombosis risk, sequential compression devices, thromboembolism-deterrent stockings, all dressing changes, hot and cold therapy, O_2, incentive spirometer, etc.?	
Did you highlight related data in similar colors in the data and interpretation section to show relationships?	

Care Plan

Nursing Diagnosis (Nursing Diagnosis Label and Related to)

Is each nursing diagnosis something you or your RN treated as the nurse caring for this patient?	
Are the top three priority nursing diagnoses listed for this patient?	
Are each of the nursing diagnosis labels highlighted in a color to match the corresponding data in your data collection?	
Have you thought about "emotional" as well as "physical" nursing diagnoses?	
Have you remembered not to use medical diagnoses in your nursing diagnostic statements?	

Supporting Data (as Evidenced by)

Are all of your supporting data on the care plan listed in your data collection? All supporting data should be from the data collection and written verbatim.	
Are the supporting data pertinent to the nursing diagnosis? Are there data missing that you should have collected related to that nursing diagnosis?	

Short-Term Goal (STG)

Is the goal realistic and patient-centered, and is the outcome you identified measurable?	
Is there a time frame for meeting the goal?	
Does the outcome of the goal relate directly to resolving the problem identified as your nursing diagnosis?	

Interventions with Rationale

Is each intervention written specifically for your patient?	
Have you listed a rationale for each of your nursing interventions?	
Does each of the rationales make sense for your patient?	
Does each of the rationales have a page citation from the text or source listed as your evidence-based practice (EBP) citation?	
Did you use your required course textbook and/or nursing diagnosis reference book for identifying rationales?	

Rational Reference(s)/EBP

Did you include an APA-style reference for the sources of your rationales?	

Evaluation

Does your evaluation indicate whether the patient met the goal?	
If so, what should be done regarding the plan of care? Should it be continued, modified, or discontinued?	
If not, what needs to change in the care plan to assist with the patient's achievement of the goal, or does the plan of care need to be discontinued and shifted to a different goal and focus?	

Final Reminder

Using various colors, be sure to highlight related data and corresponding nursing diagnostic labels in similar colors in the data collection and interpretation section, and at the top of the care plan.

APPENDIX C

Abbreviations

\# number

< less than

> greater than

≤ less than or equal to

≥ greater than or equal to

↑ increased

→ to

↓ decreased

2° secondary to

A&O alert and oriented

ABG arterial blood gas

AC or ac before meals

AD Alzheimer disease

ADA American Diabetes Association

ADL activities of daily living

AEB or aeb as evidenced by

AED automated external defibrillator

AF or Afib atrial fibrillation

AKI acute kidney injury

ALT alanine aminotransferase

AM morning

AP alkaline phosphatase

aPTT or APTT activated partial thromboplastin time

AST aspartate aminotransferase

AVF arteriovenous fistula

BID, bid, b.i.d. twice a day

BMI body mass index

BMP basic metabolic panel: sodium (Na), chloride (Cl), blood urea nitrogen (BUN), potassium (K^+), carbon dioxide (CO_2), creatinine (CR), and blood glucose (BS)

BNP brain natriuretic peptide

BP blood pressure

bpm beats per minute or breaths per minute

BS bowel sounds or blood sugar or blood glucose

BUN blood urea nitrogen

C celsius

c̄ with

C&DB cough and deep breath

Ca calcium

CA cancer

CAD coronary artery disease

CAUTI catheter-associated urinary tract infection

CBC complete blood count; white blood cells (WBC), hemoglobin (HGB), hematocrit (HCT), platelets (PLT)

CCM conceptual care map

CCU cardiac care unit

CDC Centers for Disease Control and Prevention

C-diff or C. difficile *Clostridium difficile*

CKD chronic kidney disease

Cl chloride

cm centimeter

CO_2 carbon dioxide

COCA color, odor, consistency, and amount of a fluid

COPD chronic obstructive pulmonary disease

CPR cardiopulmonary resuscitation

CR creatinine

CT computed tomography

CVA cerebrovascular accident, stroke

CVD cardiovascular disease

D_5W dextrose 5% and water

DASH dietary approaches to stop hypertension

DBP diastolic BP

DC or dc discontinue

DEXA scan dual-energy x-ray absorptiometry scan

DKA diabetic ketoacidosis

dL deciliter

DM diabetes mellitus

DNR do not resuscitate

DOE dyspnea on exertion

DVT deep vein thrombosis

EBP evidence-based practice

ECG, EKG electrocardiogram

ED emergency department

EEG electroencephalogram

EGD esophagogastroduodenoscopy

eGFR estimated glomerular filtration rate

EHR   electronic health record
EMR   electronic medical record
EMT   emergency medical technician
ER   emergency room or extended release
ESKD   end-stage kidney disease
F   Fahrenheit
FA   forearm
Fe   iron
g   gauge or gram
GI   gastrointestinal
H, h, or hr   hour
H&H   hemoglobin and hematocrit
HAI   healthcare-associated infection or hospital-acquired infection
HbA$_{1C}$ hemoglobin A$_{1C}$, glycosylated hemoglobin
HCO$_3$ bicarbonate
Hct or HCT   hematocrit
HD   hemodialysis
HDL   high-density lipoprotein
HF   heart failure
Hg   mercury
Hgb or HGB   hemoglobin
Hgb S   hemoglobin S
HOB   head of bed
HTN   hypertension
I&O   intake and output
In or in   inch
INR   international normalized ratio
IU   international unit
IV   intravenous
JVD   jugular vein distention
K$^+$ potassium
kg   kilogram
L   left or liter
Lb or lb   pounds
LBM   last bowel movement
LDL   low-density lipoprotein
LFA   left forearm
LFT   liver function tests
LH   left hand
LLQ   left lower quadrant
LMWH   low-molecular-weight heparin
LPN/LVN   licensed practical nurse/licensed vocational nurse
LUQ   left upper quadrant
m   meter
MAE   moves all extremities
MAP   mean arterial pressure
MAR   medication administration record
mcg   microgram
mEq   milliequivalent
mg   milligram
MI   myocardial infarction, heart attack
MICU   medical intensive care unit

min   minute
mL, ml   milliliter
mm   millimeter
mmol   millimole
Na   sodium
NANDA-I   NANDA International (formerly North American Nursing Diagnosis Association)
NAS   no added salt
NC   nasal cannula
NG   nasogastric
NIC   nursing interventions classification
NKDA   no known drug allergies
NOC   nursing outcomes classification
NPO   nothing by mouth
NS   normal saline
NSAID   nonsteroidal antiinflammatory drug
NSR   normal sinus rhythm
NSS   normal saline solution
N&V, n/v   nausea and vomiting
O$_2$ sat   oxygen saturation
OR   operating room
ORIF   open reduction internal fixation
OT   occupational therapy
p   after
P   pulse
PaCO$_2$ partial pressure of carbon dioxide in arterial blood
PACU   post anesthesia care unit
PaO$_2$ partial pressure of oxygen in arterial blood
PCA   patient controlled analgesia
PCN   penicillin
PCP   primary care provider, i.e., physician or nurse practitioner
PD   peritoneal dialysis
PE   pulmonary embolism
PERRLA   pupils equal, round, and reactive to light and accommodation
pg   picogram
PICC   peripherally inserted central catheter
PLT   platelets
PM   afternoon or evening
PO   by mouth
ppd   pack per day
PPE   personal protective equipment
PRN   as needed
pt or Pt   patient
PT   physical therapy
PT/INR   prothrombin time/international normalized ratio
PUD   peptic ulcer disease
Pulse ox   pulse oximetry
q   every
R   respirations or right
r/o or R/O   rule out

r/t or R/T   related to
RA   room air
RFA   right forearm
RH   right hand
RLQ   right lower quadrant
RN   registered nurse
ROM   range of motion
RT   respiratory therapy
RUQ   right upper quadrant
s̄   without
s/p, S/P   status post
SBP   systolic blood pressure
SCC   sickle cell crisis
SCD   sequential compression device or sickle cell disease
SCT   sickle cell trait
SOB   short of breath

SSRI   selective serotonin release inhibitor
STG   short-term goal
subcut   subcutaneous
T   temperature
TPN   total parenteral nutrition
Tx or tx   treatment
UAP   unlicensed assistive personnel
Up ad lib   up as desired
UTI   urinary tract infection
VS   vital signs
VT   ventricular tachycardia
VTE   venous thromboembolism
WBC   white blood cell
WNL   within normal limits
WOCN   wound ostomy continence nurse

Conceptual Care Mapping

Case Studies for Improving Communication, Collaboration, and Care

Learn to prioritize patient care quickly and effectively!

Using a "two books in one" approach, this nursing text guides you through the most important aspects of patient care and critical thinking. The first section explores the title's three C's of nursing: communication, collaboration within the health care team, and care. The second section includes case studies that progress from simple clinical conditions to the more complex, challenging you to prioritize your approach to care.

Outstanding Features

- **Conceptual Care Mapping** guides your care—using templates and an online, interactive conceptual care map creator—from the author team who developed this new method of organizing care information.

- **30 case studies** focus on the patients you are most likely to see in clinical experience and teach you to think critically.

- **Elsevier's Conceptual Care Map (CCM) creator** helps you create, update, manage, and submit care maps quickly and effectively.

- **Answers and completed care maps** are provided for selected cases to reinforce what you've learned.

- **Interprofessional education and collaboration** are key elements in all of the case studies, helping you understand how you will work within the larger health care team.

Recommended
Shelving Classifications
Nursing Fundamentals
Medical-Surgical
Nursing

ISBN 978-0-323-48037-6

9 780323 480376

ELSEVIER   elsevier.com

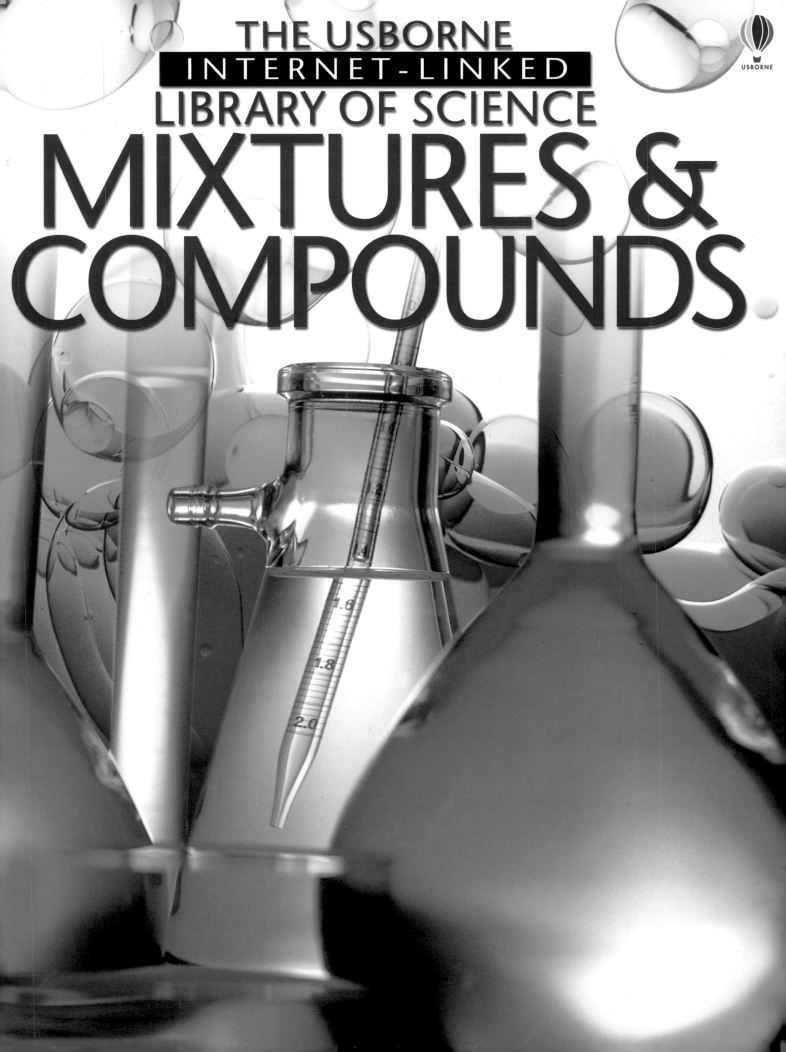

THE USBORNE
INTERNET-LINKED
LIBRARY OF SCIENCE
MIXTURES &
COMPOUNDS